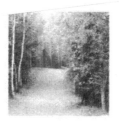

Our
Road Back

A Collection of Personal Accounts from Patients
with Connective Tissue Diseases
Treated with Antibiotic Therapies

Various Authors

Compiled by
Hanna Rhee, MD

This book is sold at cost.
No profit is made from the purchase of this book.
Price is set based on production, publication, and
advertisement avenue for this book.

Front Cover Photo:
Eden Lake, Alaska

Our Road Back

Disclaimer

Any and all statements made by authors regarding their medical conditions and subsequent care or lack thereof have *not* been verified against their respective medical records, treating entities, organizations, physicians, or other parties or individuals mentioned in their respective accounts. Perspectives written by authors are considered to be their own opinions and are *not* necessarily the opinion of any individual or party associated with the compilation or publication of this book.

This book is *not* meant in any way to offer medical advice including but not limited to evaluation, diagnosis and treatment in regards to the reader's own medical condition nor to suggest or imply the unverified treatment options stated by authors will be effective for other patients. *No* individual or party associated with the compilation or publication of this book is stating, suggesting, nor implying any statements in this book be used to replace a visit to the reader's own healthcare provider. Readers are reminded that medications or other treatment options may cause *adverse* side effects in certain individuals. Readers are therefore strongly encouraged to discuss their medical condition and treatment options with their own healthcare providers.

TABLE OF CONTENTS

ACKNOWLEDGMENTS

Dr. & Lenee' Sinnott
For their kindness and endless support
in the compilation of this book

Bev & Dave
For their indispensible assistance and warmth
through the bitter cold of winter

ia'kona
For his forgiveness
in leaving Hawai'i

Barney
For lending his fur
so that others may stay warm, too

Our Road Back

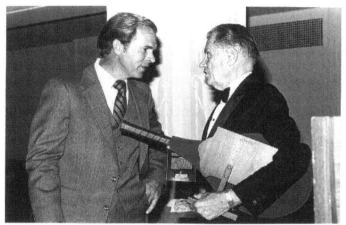

Thomas McPherson Brown, MD (R)
John S. Sinnott, DO (L)

*Of those
who came before us...*

Our Road Back

*Dedicated
to those in search
of their own
Road Back
home...*

Our
Road Back

1

From Alaska to Ida Grove

The buffalo were knocking our fence down again, and it was up to me to stop them. What a frustrating, labor intensive chore to mend fence. My patience with these wild creatures had grown thin. Everything in my life had become so difficult, so overwhelming. Daily chores of chopping wood and hauling water pushed me to the limit. Every part of my body HURT, and I had no idea why. It seemed like muscle strain that would never heal itself. I couldn't sit for any length of time, walking was painful, and I couldn't sleep. The summer of 2010 was MISERABLE.

Here I was, living my lifelong dream and hating life! My husband and I spent the last 15 years working to establish a wilderness retreat to cater to disabled hunters. Deep in the Alaskan bush, the nearest single lane dirt road is 50 miles away, accessible only in the winter when the river is frozen. Getting to a doctor was out of the question.

A lightening strike this spring started a raging 50,000 acre wildfire. It was within a mile of our ranch before the rains came and detoured it around us. At the same time, the motor in our bush plane ceased to work, leaving my husband and I separated for the summer. Him in town, me alone at the Ranch. Stress level was high.

We have a small herd of buffalo and a small herd of Norwegian Fjord horses that I'm responsible for. There were 50 acres of hay that needed to be cut, baled and stacked. Normally this is what I thrived on. But this summer, my mysterious state of physical pain kept me in tears and in a state of dread. I was taking 12 ibuprofens a day and still had a difficult time moving. The thought of getting on a horse was out of the question. I could only "pull" myself up a flight of stairs, one at a time. I could not turn my head to the right or the left. I could not open my mouth wide enough to use a fork. Getting dressed and undressed was agonizing. In bed, I would lie awake and cry.

Midway through September, my husband rescued me and flew me to town for a doctor visit. It was so difficult to climb into that little bush plane and just as difficult to get into our truck. No part of my body would work. At 55 years of age, I equaled myself to a 90 year old. I was quickly on my way to being completely crippled. Blood tests were done and three days later I received an email from the Fairbanks doctor saying "Your labs look like you are developing Rheumatoid Arthritis or one of its variants. There are two medications I want you to start on, prednisone and methotrexate."

What the heck did that mean????? We have lived without running water or electricity for years, but we do have an expensive satellite internet system and that was just about to pay for itself. First I googled Rheumatoid Arthritis and was in shock and disbelief by what I read --- "can destroy

2

organs"?!?!?! The second search was for methotrexate. I thought it must be a joke. WHY would I take that??? My homework was just beginning. I spent countless hours reading everything I could on the disease and treatments. It seemed like I kept reading the same stuff over and over. There was no way out!

I finally gave in to the pain and started on the prednisone. The doctor changed his mind about the methotrexate and started me on [name brand] hydroxychloroquine. I was so depressed to think I had to take these "poison meds". My homework continued. When I was on my fifth day of taking [name brand] hydroxychloroquine with nightmares of vision loss, I happened across a short little blip on the internet where someone, somewhere, mentioned "go to *The Road Back Foundation* (RBF) website to read about antibiotic treatment." I wish with all my heart that I could thank that unknown writer. "Whoever" had instantly changed my life from HOPELESS to HOPEFUL. The fun was just about to begin.

The RBF website is full of priceless information… an oasis in the desert. The volunteers and members are very helpful. They have answers that I could not find anywhere else. What a support system!!! I had a strong sense that I would not be finding the medical help I needed in Alaska. Bouncing from doctor to doctor until finding one that would really help was not in our budget. I had noticed the name "Dr. S" mentioned several times on the site. An RBF member told me she knew of no doctor in my area, but she would highly recommend Dr. SINNOTT in Iowa. Now I had a name and a state… but Iowa???? I blew the dust off my atlas. I got his email address and sent him a quick note: "Are you taking new patients?" His response was fast and short. "Yes, and we have an opening Thanksgiving week." I quickly accepted.

Asking the Fairbanks doctor for a referral to go to Iowa seemed to infuriate him and his answer was a definite "NO". That meant I would not be getting any financial help from our insurance. My sense was strong that I HAD to go... this was my ONLY hope. I started making reservations. Airline, motel and car for a week... it added up fast. My dear husband would fly me from the Ranch to the airport but the weather forecast called for snow. That meant he would have to take me to town and drop me off two days early so as to not miss my flight. That meant two days at a motel.

The flight from Fairbanks to Anchorage was ON TIME!!!!
The flight from Anchorage to Seattle was ON TIME!!!!

The flight from Seattle to Minneapolis was delayed indefinitely due to snow and ice. Oh oh. And worse than that my flight to Sioux City had been cancelled. The clock was ticking... I had an appointment I had to keep!! Thirty-eight hours of airport later, I was wearily standing at the rental care counter in Sioux City, Iowa. I would make it to Ida Grove with ten hours to spare before my appointment. Checking into the Ida Grove hotel was like entering heaven. A bed, hot running water, electricity, and television. Such luxury. I was on vacation now.

The Monday morning appointment went well. The hospital in Ida Grove is new and easy to navigate through. The office staff was quick to take care of all the paperwork. I then met The Doctor that I had traveled over 3,500 miles to see. I was not disappointed. Dr. Sinnott entered the room with a young, attractive lady wearing medical scrubs. He introduced us, saying that she a doctor from Hawai'i visiting Ida Grove to do some research on AP with him. That was great news to me... doctors we are so badly in need of. Dr. Sinnott answered all my questions and explained the therapy to me. He then turned me over to the nurses that are in charge of administering the IV's.

4

With the hospital being open 24 hours a day, it works out real slick that you can choose what time you want to receive the twice a day IVs administered at least six hours apart. One IV in the early morning and the second IV in the evening leaves the whole day available to explore the town and surrounding area. I'd consider Ida Grove a good vacation spot. The only thing the town lacks is a S_ coffeehouse or anything that resembles a S_. THAT was a bummer.

On Thanksgiving morning I met with Dr. Sinnott again. He gave me my test results and the prescriptions that I would be needing. Two more IVs and I would be free to return to Alaska. Can it really be this simple?? Looking back a few years, I can see that my unexplained fatigue was not in my imagination, but the first sign of RA. My fatigue disappeared the same time the inflammation went away. A full night's sleep returned after being absent for years.

Today it is 40 degree below zero in Alaska. I got my chores done, buffalo fed, horses watered and enough wood stacked to keep the stove going. It's easy to get dressed and climb stairs again. I'm not 100% yet, but it's only been 2½ months since my journey to Iowa. I'm well on my way to full recovery... AP WORKS. I'm really looking forward to working with the horses and riding this spring.

The most important things on this detour of life have been that I did not rely on this Alaskan doctor's direction of toxic meds and hopelessness. I thank God daily for the ability to heal. I'm thankful for a loving, supportive spouse who carried my workload when I could not (He has since installed an indoor toilet - wow!). I'm especially thankful for *The Road Back Foundation* and Dr. Sinnott for going against mainstream medicine and providing AP to us. I would not hesitate to make that long trip to Ida Grove again. Life is good.

Thank you Dr. Sinnott,
M.P.

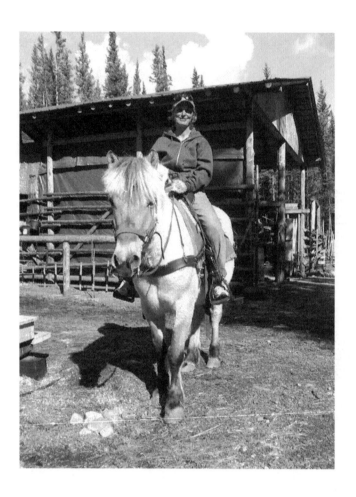

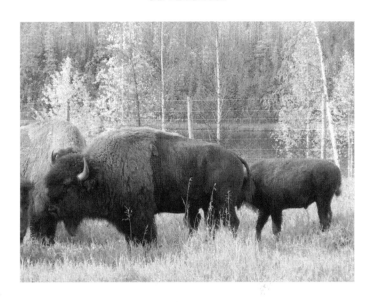

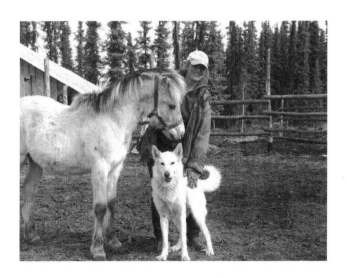

Our Road Back

2

Antibiotic Therapy:
Relief without Worry

Rheumatoid arthritis (RA) first made its appearance in my life in 1972 when I was 30 years old. I used to like to tell people I went to bed feeling fine and woke up with RA. I woke up with severe, unrelenting pain at the base of my thumb. It eventually went away only to return several weeks later in the opposite hand in the exact same place. I later learned this was typical. I find it interesting that prior to this, I had a viral infection of some kind as others had also reported this prior to the onset of RA.

I went to a doctor, and she performed a number of tests. By this time, the pain had moved to numerous joints. She suspected RA and started me on a regimen of 15 aspirins a day. When that proved to be ineffective, she then started me on gold shots. I wasn't too happy about this since I knew it could affect several organs in my body, and I had urine and blood tests regularly. I believe the gold shots worked for approximately 10 years. Next, the doctor discussed several

9

meds including methotrexate. I knew immediately that was one I would try to avoid. Instead, I chose [name brand] hydroxychloroquine, which could "only" damage your eyes. That drug finally became ineffective after about seven years. In the meantime, I happened to be at the library browsing the nonfiction shelves and discovered <u>The Road Back</u> by Dr. Brown. I read that book cover to cover at once! It just made such good sense to me. I figured if it could work on a gorilla, why not on me?

It took quite a while to find a doctor that offered antibiotic therapy. I finally found one near Chicago. He started me on the therapy, and I did feel worse before improving, but not as badly as anticipated. Relatives, friends, and even doctors really did not believe I would have any success with this rather "simple" form of therapy. But I did, and I'm happy to say it worked on me for 12 years without having to worry about any horrible side effects.

When the antibiotics became less and less effective, I went to see Dr. Sinnott in Ida Grove, Iowa. The doctor was kind and compassionate as were the rest of the staff at the clinic and hospital. We stayed for almost a week, and I received infusions. I did feel somewhat better for a while, but eventually it quit working altogether. I did try one more round of infusions but it was just never the same.

I went back to [name brand] hydroxychloroquine for a while and am now on [name brand] leflunomide and 5 mg of prednisone. I am once again worrying about toxic damage to my body. I guess I'll have to make another trip to Ida Grove.

Judith J.
Wisconsin

3

An Answer to Prayer

Hi to all who read this! Where do I begin, or how do I start so it's interesting to other readers? When I first heard about this book of folks who experienced Dr. Sinnott's antibiotic treatments, I was excited to say the least. But I thought there'd probably be lots of other people who will write their story that they probably wouldn't miss mine if I didn't send one. But with encouragement from my dear husband and our parents, I decided to write one anyway and to do my best!

I married Johnny Sept 19, 2002. Around that time we knew something was not right with me. We suspected Lyme disease (LD) as I remembered finding a tick on me while working at the greenhouse. We knew so little about Lyme, so I ended up taking lots of herbs and just lived with it. In November 2003, we were blessed with our little boy Edwin. He wasn't more than a week old when I started getting ill. I hurt so bad I wouldn't wish it on anyone else. I swallowed lots of painkillers just so I can bare it. Then, we packed up and went to an LD specialist in Pennsylvania that someone had recommended to us. He said I had Lyme and rheumatoid arthritis. His treatments did help somewhat, but it just brought me so far and that's where I stayed. So we lost our faith in that doctor and went to one in Maryland. He could not find any LD but said I had RA and sent me home to find a doctor closer to where we lived. Now this doc also informed us that everyone that goes to the LD specialist is diagnosed with LD, so there's a question of whether I ever had it in the first place! Well, I was also not interested in seeing docs in town because I didn't want all those bad pain medications, but I learned to take naproxen which helped.

In 2005, we decided to go to Mexico. There they gave me medications that made me feel so good I could work more, walk better, etc. The medicine wasn't supposed to have side effects, but I know it made me hungry and gave me chipmunk cheeks. But hey, I could live with that if they helped me feel so much better. Then in 2008 I got pregnant again, and it was a drag. The doctors had told me some women with RA wanted to be pregnant. Well, not this one. But I am very glad we have two healthy children! Then in June 2009, we were blessed with a little girl named Lydiann. We just couldn't believe how good I felt the first few weeks after the baby was born. I could take care of her and even nurse her, but that soon changed. I ached and hurt so bad that people came and took care of my baby, something that was really hard for me to accept. So we once again started searching for something that helped. We decided to give Mexico another try. There they gave me chelation therapy and a stem cell transplant, but I just didn't get much help from it.

Soon after we came home from Mexico, I got a note from a friend about a woman name Judy Cash and her phone number. This woman had found lots of help getting treated in Iowa. So my dad called her up, and it sounded too good to be true. We got in contact with another Amish couple that was there, and they also highly recommended Dr. Sinnott's antibiotic treatments. So in April of 2010, my parents went with me to Ida Grove, Iowa. Well, first of all we were so taken with the friendly people of Ida Grove. Being Amish, we didn't know how they would take to us, but there weren't any problems. We became friends with Dr. Sinnott and his other patients. We got to know Judy Cash very well and spent a fun week together.

I did my ten IV treatments then headed home not knowing what to expect. But let me tell you: it's the best thing we've ever done for my RA. It's such a blessing not to hurt and hurt. Now I don't feel worse every time the weather changes. I still take some pain pills but not as many as before. I hope with time, I can stop taking them. My hands are crippled quite a bit and were very painful, but not anymore. Today, I can walk and use my hands much better. Mopping floors was always my hubby's job, but now I can do it myself. I'm even looking forward to gardening this year!

I've now done my second round of IV treatments and feel it was worthwhile. After my treatments, I went through a slump which was expected. But since I'm over that, I feel better than I have in years. So we believe getting to know about Dr. Sinnott was an answer to prayer. Yes, we feel it's the way to go and we highly recommend Dr. Sinnott to anyone with what some call an autoimmune disease. I'll gladly give more information if someone is interested.

Wishing you all God's Richest Blessings,

Mrs. Miriam E. Mast
8237 N. Lighthouse Lane
Opdyke, IL 62872

Our Road Back

4

"My" Road Back from Ida Grove

My name is Judy Cash, and I am one of Dr. Sinnott's success stories. I was diagnosed with Rheumatoid Arthritis in April of 2009, but my story began a few years earlier. In 2002, my mother passed away very suddenly. She had come to my house to recover from a hospital stay. While there, she was doing well but upon awakening the day before Christmas, she fell to the floor and was gone. I was in shock and had a very difficult time with this. She was my rock, my stability. She was my best friend. We had also just bought a house and were in the process of moving when my mom got sick. I believe this is part of the stress that brought on my symptoms.

Then around 2004-2005, I started feeling very tired and had little energy. I also began having what I called "sick spells" where I would be fine one minute and the next minute I was trembling and weak, sick to my stomach, and my heart would be pounding and seem to skip beats. I felt as if I would collapse if I didn't lie down. I tried eating something, thinking it was low blood sugar, but it didn't help. The only relief I got was lying still and taking a short nap. I would also check my blood pressure which was usually low. These symptoms continued until I started this treatment. My blood work was always normal, and my doctor said it was depression or a lack of sleep. Then I began having more trouble than usual with my ankles. I would be walking fine then turn my ankle or fall on level ground or in parking lots for no reason. I fell so many times; I can't even begin to count the number of times. Once I fell in our barn and turned my ankle. I was unable to get up by myself, but luckily my two children were there since I was unable to walk at all. The pain was severe, and I became afraid of what was happening to me.

Things got worse. I began having very severe pain in different parts of my body, hands, fingers, wrists, palms, upper arms, shoulders, knees, lower legs, feet and toes. At times my muscles were so weak; I was unable to reach my arms up to put dishes in the cabinet. If I used my hands for anything, the next day I would be unable to move them at all. I'd have to just sit and hold my hands very still and cry because the pain was so severe. I used wrist braces on both hands, especially when driving, just to stabilize them. I could hardly walk. I tried many different insoles, but they didn't give me much relief. My doctor sent me to an orthopedic specialist who said my toe pain was caused by a hammer toe. He suggested a toe straightener which gave me some relief.

The symptoms were happening so fast that I couldn't keep up with them. I was scared to confide in others and kept a lot of this to myself. Depression began creeping in, and I started forgetting things. My children noticed this more than anyone else. They often laughed at me for saying the wrong words or going blank in the middle of talking or doing something. It was getting really bad for me. I was embarrassed and even thought I must be losing my mind. I felt so alone and thought no one could possibly understand what I was going through. I felt hopeless, but I wanted to find a solution. Every night I was reading on the internet, trying to connect all my symptoms.

I also began having tingling in my hands and feet, and I was referred to a neurologist. All my tests came back fine. He believed it was some type of arthritis. I was then sent to an arthritis specialist, who said she was not sure of my diagnosis but was not convinced it was RA.

One evening while grocery shopping, I began to feel so terrible in the store that I could only scoot my feet across the floor. I wasn't sure I could even go through the checkout and get home. I prayed for the strength to just get home safely. I cried all the way home and prayed to the Lord to point me in the right direction, to find the solution that would help me. I had two young children that I had to raise, and I was having a hard time coping with everything.

When I got home, I went straight to my computer even though my hands and feet were hurting terribly, but I was desperate to find a solution. I read everything I thought might help, skipping around on different sites, finally ending on the Rheumatic Support website and from there, I found *The Road Back* site. This was the first time I felt hopeful. I was so excited that I could hardly wait until morning to tell someone what I had found. The information about autoimmune diseases being caused by *Mycoplasma* and being treated with antibiotics just made sense to me. I wanted to believe it and I did, with all my heart. After contacting Dr. Sinnott in Ida Grove, Iowa I was further convinced I could be helped with this treatment. About the same time, I finally received my diagnosis of RA. In June of 2009, several years after all my problems started, my family and I were on our way to Ida Grove. The trip was over 700 miles one way. It was such a pleasure to meet and be treated by Dr. Sinnott who was the first doctor who truly took an interest in me and my health. He spent time with me asking and answering questions about my medical issues. He prescribed antibiotics by IV twice a day for five days. On my last day there, I met with Dr. Sinnott again. He gave me such encouragement toward my recovery. I left Ida Grove feeling hopeful.

After returning home and getting my prescription for minocycline filled, I began feeling worse than I had ever felt before. I could barely function. One day I could not even get out of bed or walk by myself. Another day I needed help getting dressed because I was unable to lift my arms. I figured it was the Herxheimer effect which was a good sign that the antibiotics were working. Yet, I was concerned.

I noticed the label on the medicine bottle did not say minocycline. I called the pharmacy and talked with them. They realized that they had given me the wrong medicine; I had already taken it for two weeks. I immediately called Dr. Sinnott who told me to get started on the minocycline and that the mix-up was likely the reason I felt so bad. He felt everything would be fine. It took about four more weeks before I began to feel better, and I continued improving weekly. Soon I could tell a big difference. The severe pain I had at the beginning of my illness was gone and to this day, I have never had the severe pain again. I did continue to feel some fatigue and weakness at times, but that gradually got better too.

After about ten months on minocycline, I felt I might benefit from another week of IV's. Dr. Sinnott also thought it could give me another boost, so I was on my way to Ida Grove once again. I believe the treatment was successful even though I didn't see a big difference right away as I'd experienced after my first IV's. Then after about two months or so, I began to feel like my old self again before I was sick. I have to this day continued to improve.

It has been one year and eight months since I began my treatment. Even though it's been a very difficult journey in my life and I lost a few years that I can never get back, I have never regretted my decision to go with this treatment. I would hate to imagine where I would be today if I had not been able to use the internet and find *The Road Back* and Dr. Sinnott. I have received many calls from people who, by word of mouth, have heard of my success using the antibiotic treatment. I have and will continue to send people to Ida Grove and Dr. Sinnott.

In closing, I would like to say thank you to Dr. Sinnott and for all that he does for people every day. He is truly a remarkable man who gives of his time and genuinely cares about his patients' health and wellbeing. In today's society, this is a rare quality. I have my life back because of him, and I am very grateful! I want to thank the Rheumatic Support team and *The Road Back* team for their time and support. I am also grateful for them! I also want to thank my family and dear friends who stood by me with loving support and encouragement during my darkest days. I could not have made it through without all their love and prayers. Most of all...

I thank my Lord
for
guiding my way
on
My Road Back

I will be glad to talk to anyone about this treatment. You may call me at 606-758-8077.

Judy

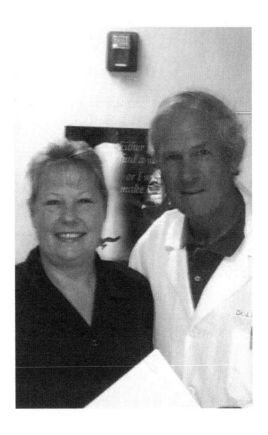

5

My Mom's Road Back

From time to time
I think about the things
my mom went through.
It makes me sad
because I didn't have a clue.
She went through pain
unbearable,
pain no one could understand.
The pain was often
in her feet or hands.
She had no one to turn to,
or look to for support.
She decided to search the internet
for anything
to explain her pain.
She found The Road Back website
and the people who understood.
They told her of Dr. Sinnott,
and the love and care he gave.
(continued)

21

We packed up and went to Iowa
and stayed there for a week.
She took a round of IV's.
When we were on our way back home,
you may not believe,
my mom climbed
from the front seat of the van
then into the center
and felt no pain.
I have written many poems,
but this one is not the same,
it is not about
a bird or a plane,
it is about my mom
and the things she went through
with
RA.

Rachel Cash
(age 13)

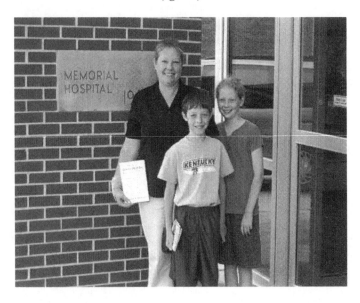

6

My Antibiotic Therapy Experience

My affliction, Polymyalgia Rheumatica, started slowly in mid-May 2006. My right ear ached slightly, sounded like fluid in my ear, and then my teeth started aching on that side. My family doctor said my ears were clear, maybe TMJ? He advised me to rest my jaw, apply ice or heat, whichever felt better, then take some [name brand] acetaminophen. My husband and I went to northern Wisconsin where I had trouble chewing. I found several wood ticks on me, but my ailment had started before that.

<u>May 26, 2006</u>
I got up during the night because my jaw and teeth hurt enough to wake me. I took [name brand] acetaminophen and a cold cloth helped some. These symptoms continued on and off for several days.

June 1-2, 2006

We were in Storm Lake, Iowa at a family reunion. I had problems talking and chewing. Both tired me out. When we returned to our recreation center in Cedar Rapids, I had a physical therapist examine me. She didn't think it was TMJ, maybe poor posture. She gave me exercises which didn't help. Our daughter is a chiropractor. She gave me several treatments which didn't help my symptoms. I slept propped up, and I changed pillows but nothing helped.

June 15, 2006

I talked to a group one evening about renewable energy. My jaw and throat were very "tired" after all that talking. Same symptoms for the next few days. I took [name brand] acetaminophen and its PM version to help me sleep.

June 19, 2006

I began to hurt all over, sudden hip and knee pain, shooting pains in my head, all my teeth ached, and then my temples felt swollen and sore. I couldn't touch them or lie down. Family doctor sent me to a lab for several tests. Sed test elevated, Lyme disease negative. I was in agony for the next few days. I couldn't touch my head, up most of the night taking [name brand] acetaminophen, rocking and crying in a recliner.

June 23, 2006

The family doctor diagnosed me with PMR. He was worried about Temporal Arteritis (TA). He prescribed 60 mg of prednisone a day and recommended arterial biopsy ASAP, which was scheduled for July 5th. I went off my warfarin in preparation for surgery, but continued on a baby aspirin per day. Then I caught a bad head cold, up most nights, really miserable, coughing, congested, and worried. Touch and go if I should have the biopsy, but I did. The surgeon took 2 inch piece of artery from my temples. Results were negative. I started back on warfarin (also had taken [name brand] digoxin for decades).

Prednisone eased the pains, but did a job on me in other ways. I was so jittery and "high" all the time. I crashed every day about mid-day and slept soundly for a couple hours. I ate all the time, even got up during the night to eat, but lost 10 lbs. instead of gaining weight. I normally avoid fast food, but craved their fish sandwiches and coffee! Luckily, I did not have a "moon face". Prednisone at 60 mg didn't seem to last through the night, so my family doctor reluctantly upped it to 80 mg/day with the warning that he wanted me off of it ASAP because of negative side effects.

I was really "wired" on that much prednisone and very worried about my bones (my mom had severe osteoporosis and suffered terribly). I acted irrationally, shopping sprees for unneeded items, even ended up with a "free" 135 lb dog (Akita mix) someone was giving away, over my husband's strong objections. Up and down all night, cleaning drawers, sorting papers. I couldn't sit still enough to read or write day or night. Doctor advised cutting back on prednisone by 10 mg/wk, but that was too quick. I had what I thought were "withdrawals". It felt like what I've read DTs are: violent shaking, wild thoughts.

Over many weeks of trial and error, I found I could only cut back 2.5 mg/week. I tired easily, couldn't take the heat at all. I had to let my beautiful garden go to weeds. Very depressing. I feel like I lost a whole year of my life.

One of my brothers encouraged me to talk to his older son Mike in Erie, Pennsylvania who had been diagnosed with Rheumatoid Arthritis eight years earlier. He had been taking strong drugs until his aunt, a nurse, told him he was taking chemotherapy drugs which would not cure him, but might kill him.

The mother of Mike's wrestling buddy had also been diagnosed with RA. She went to Dr. John Sinnott for antibiotic therapy, was doing very well, in remission, and taking few if any drugs. Mike started with Dr. Sinnott and with good results. He and I have kept in touch about our afflictions. He says "Dr. Sinnott saved my life Aunt Bev. Go see him."

My husband and I drove to Ida Grove and stayed in the motel near the hospital. I got the IV treatment and then was put on minocycline 100 mg twice a day. I did not have the Herxheimer effect. I chose a room with a tub so I could soak in Epsom salts which helped a little. I ate yogurt each noon to replenish good bacteria.

I stayed on minocycline successfully for 4-1/2 years until my face started turning black, a side effect of prolonged use of minocycline. Dr. Sinnott changed me to doxycycline, but it didn't seem to do the job or else something else in my system had changed.

March-April, 2010

I thought I had had a stroke or something serious. I became so exhausted at times, during which time I couldn't talk, type or think clearly. I went to the family doctor who referred me to a neurologist in case I was developing Parkinson's or Myasthenia Gravis. The neurologist examined me thoroughly. He even did reflex testing. He didn't think I had had a stroke, and I didn't exhibit symptoms of Parkinson's or Myasthenia Gravis either. He doesn't believe in Antibiotic Therapy, "unproven" is what he said. Maybe sleep apnea? I asked Dr. Sinnott if these symptoms could be associated with PMR. He said patients had complained of "brain fog" but not trouble speaking.

I had two sleep tests which showed mild sleep apnea. The neurologist felt because I have atrial fibrillation, it might be good to use a CPAP (continuous positive airway pressure) machine. I started that mid-May 2010, but instead of decreasing the number of times I stopped breathing, my rate went way up, which stymied the neurologist and sleep therapist. I kept using the machine and got the instances way down, but discontinued use when the weather turned cold (we have no heat upstairs in our bedroom). I will resume when the weather warms up, although I didn't notice any discernable difference at first. Now I'm starting to get the exhaustion/speech problem occasionally.

Late summer, 2010

I began aching and hurting again, slight earache, fluid sounds, jaw ache. In December, Dr. Sinnott prescribed azithromycin 250 mg M-W-F for a two month trial, but so far nothing has improved. I have gotten several adjustments and massages during the winter, which felt good at the time, but didn't relieve my symptoms long term.

As a result of seeing Dr. Sinnott, any time I mention something about my PMR affliction to my family doctor, he tells me that I am "under the care of another physician for that." Early on I gave him an information sheet about Antibiotic Therapy and asked if he wanted to be part of my treatment, but he didn't. He does not believe it's a proven treatment. This makes it very awkward for me because I, the patient, have to diagnose whether something that's happening, like my ears/jaw exhaustion, is part of my affliction or something else. I can't talk to him about it. I can't really consult Dr. Sinnott about something not related to my PMR since he is retired except for rheumatic patients. I do not like not knowing who to talk to.

Any doctor to whom I have mentioned Antibiotic Therapy always says the same thing, "there haven't been enough studies, and it's not proven to be effective." So it isn't that they haven't heard of it, it's just that they have been discouraged from taking it seriously or using Antibiotic Therapy.

April 2011

I asked Dr. Sinnott to go back on low dose prednisone (5 mg), because I was getting to the point I could hardly get up and down out of a chair and had constant pain in my legs and shoulders. I've been taking it for a week now and see a slight improvement.

Because of the terrible weather we've had this spring, I haven't been able to get out and walk like I normally do. I hope that will change soon. We will be selling our farm and moving to a house in Marion, Iowa soon. We bought a house that has everything I NEED on one floor, washer/dryer, bathrooms, which will be an improvement over where we are now.

Yes, I would consider IV clindamycin again, but it's very difficult to have it done in Ida Grove. It means we drive all that way, stay in a motel, eat all our meals out, and have to arrange for someone to take care of our big dog... I have a call in to a hospital nearby about a special area they have for "continuing care" where they list it as "long term IV therapy." I don't know if IV Antibiotic Therapy treatment would fit their criteria, but it's worth a call. No one has responded yet...

<u>June 2011</u>
I finally received a call from a gentleman at the nearby hospital who will be helping to coordinate my IV treatments nearby so I won't have to leave town. I don't mind going to Ida Grove again and seeing Dr. Sinnott, but we're in the middle of moving out of our farmhouse into another home and just have to stay in town.

bhannon@bhannon.com
Iowa

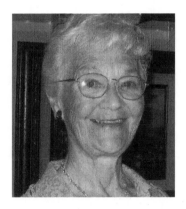

Our Road Back

7

I Have My Life Back!

About three years ago I was diagnosed with RA by a local rheumatologist. She recommended starting me on methotrexate and also needing to get monthly blood tests to monitor my liver for damage--she said this was the "gold standard" of treatment. Something seemed wrong with the medicine being almost worse than the disease, so I started looking into alternative treatments out there.

I feel so fortunate to have come across The New Arthritis Breakthrough by Henry Scammell along with some other information that confirmed this type of treatment with antibiotics was so successful--to actually treat the CAUSE of the problem and not merely treat the symptoms was such a common sense approach.

The chronic pain was almost unbearable at that time. Here I was only 50 years old and felt like I was 90! I could not walk the stairs easily, and getting in and out of a car was excruciating. I could not squeeze hard enough to use a manual can opener, turn on lamps, and turn the car key in the ignition, etc. because it was so painful. I kept saying, "I'm too young to be this old!"

By the time I made an appointment to come to Ida Grove and get treated, I was desperate to relieve the pain. The thought of living the rest of my life this way was unbearable. I was on 2,400 mg of ibuprofen daily and that only barely took the edge off. Fortunately, since we caught this fairly early, Dr. Sinnott was optimistic that I had a good chance for some relief.

I went to Ida Grove, Iowa in June 2008 for the week-long IV clindamycin treatment as an outpatient. It was probably seven months or so before I started really noticing I was getting better, but since that time I have slowly and steadily improved. As I got better, I was slowly able to wean myself off of the ibuprofen and now am completely off of it! The only medicine I take now is the minocycline twice a day.

It has been a little over 2-1/2 years since I went to Dr. Sinnott for initial treatment and I can safely say that I am now about 95 to 97% back to where I was before I was diagnosed with RA! I know there was some initial joint damage done that is irreversible but every month I have more mobility and feel like a "normal" person again!

I can confidently say this: RA is a non-factor now in my life and does not stop me from doing most things I want to do. I still have to use some moderation in certain things at times, but for the most part, it's like I am back to living life the way I used to before I was diagnosed. This has been such an answer to prayer for me and a Godsend, and I am so grateful to be able to testify that this type of treatment really works, despite what "mainstream medicine" may think and believe. I have remembered often what Dr. Sinnott told me when I first visited with him that sometimes his hardest job is to convince people to stay on the medicine because they get to feeling so much better they think they don't need it anymore. I never want to go back to how it was before and am so thankful that I don't have to. This has been one of the biggest blessings in my life, and I would like to encourage everyone reading this that this treatment really works, and I want to get the word out! It breaks my heart to see people living in such crippling pain and agony when they don't have to. I will be forever grateful for the relief from pain--I have my life back now!

Cindy C.
Leawood, Kansas

Our Road Back

8

My Miracle

I think about Dr. Sinnott and his staff often and am forever grateful for his work with antibiotic treatment. I first discovered <u>The Road Back</u> and <u>The New Arthritis Breakthrough</u> books at our local library in search for an answer to my rheumatoid arthritis that struck in 2000. It all began with strep throat and after a course of antibiotics, I thought I was fine, but about 3 weeks post-infection, my foot was swollen and looked infected. So after more antibiotics, my foot was healed, but every joint in my body was swollen, and I could barely move. This went on for months.

At the time, I had three young children and was in excruciating pain every day and wondered how I could take care of my children. I was put on a number of harsh medications by a rheumatologist that only masked my symptoms and was told I would end up in a wheelchair and that I should "just accept this and quit being depressed about my circumstances."

That was my last visit to that rheumatologist.

At first, I thought that I would just have to accept this as my life, but after an agonizing year of pain and pill popping, I sought out alternative therapy. With the encouragement of two of my nurse friends, I headed west to a well known clinic in Arizona where I spent a week to find a name to my ailment: Post Strep Reactive Arthritis. They told me it would alleviate itself over time, but there was really no time frame to go by and so for another year, I dealt with the same level of pain and discomfort.

Knowing that I could not live like this, I decided to head to the library one evening to find an answer and that is when I found "the books". I cherish these books! I had found an answer to my prayers. After reading the books, I phoned Dr. Sinnott, and he felt as if he could help me. What a blessing! So, a week before Christmas in 2002 (I think), I ventured to Ida Grove to receive treatment. Although things got worse before they got better, I stuck to the minocycline treatment and over the next few months found relief and have been in remission ever since.

I have had two more children and am active, active, active. I am forever grateful for this treatment and know that without this, I would have inevitably ended up in a wheelchair not able to enjoy the life that was given back to me by Dr. Sinnott and his staff. Thank you for continuing in this therapy as it will help so many who are suffering. I know I have been tremendously blessed and will be forever grateful for this treatment.

Sincerely,
D. Adams

9

A Lifetime
(Almost)
with Rheumatoid Arthritis

Being born and raised in Minneapolis, Minnesota was a good thing for me. It shares a border with Iowa, where over fifty years later I would be a patient of Dr. Sinnott in Iowa. We were nine people in my family, my parents and seven siblings, of which I was the middle one. My memories are mostly good, the most important being that God was invited into our home and family, and He became the Anchor in my life. He proved to be the very One I needed so much in future years.

I was in third or fourth grade when I developed scoliosis and a seventeen year old senior in high school when I got rheumatoid arthritis. Some doctors thought it may have been juvenile rheumatoid arthritis. It started in my feet and before graduation it had gone into my hands. Today it has been over fifty years that I have had the disease.

Ironically, the first doctor I went to in Minneapolis put me on antibiotics. It was in 1960-61, and I don't remember the name of it. I moved to California in the fall after graduation, and as a teenager I wasn't consistent about taking medications and just wanted the arthritis to go away.

Of course, the arthritis progressed. Through a friend whose mother had severe rheumatoid arthritis, I heard about and began a high-dose vitamin C therapy, injections and oral. After a couple of years I began going to an arthritis clinic because it was more affordable for me at the time since I was single. It was at a major hospital, and I went there for the next 8-10 years. It was there that the guessing game began as to what would be the most effective treatment for me: 12-14 aspirins daily, gold shots, prednisone, and others. Also, they did joint injections to remove fluid and inject cortisone. I saw a different doctor each month at the clinic, and my treatment would get changed according to what that particular doctor thought would work better.

I got married at age 28 and had two children, our daughter first and our son born two years later. My husband and children are and have been wonderful blessings in my life. While our son was still an infant I changed doctors and started having surgeries. It was affordable now that I was married. And for the next 27 years, I had approximately six joint related surgeries (joint replacements and fusions) while being on a regimen of gold shots, [name brand] naproxen (later [name brand] celecoxib), and methotrexate the last few years on that treatment program.

I came to realize that this treatment wasn't going to stop the progression of the arthritis because as other joints became involved surgery would be necessary again. To avoid confusion in not knowing what else to do I stayed with this treatment for many years.

After a severe reaction to medications and at the same time hearing, through a friend, about Dr. Sinnott in Iowa and his treatment using antibiotics I was ready, willing, and WANTED to try this "new" therapy. I believe it was God's timing and plan, allowing me to really "hear" my friend's recommendation and to act on it, and I made the appointment with Dr. Sinnott. I have been on this treatment for eleven years now and it has been the most effective one for me so far. The first three months I felt terrible, but I had gone off all the other medications, and I knew I was going to give the antibiotics a good try. I have confidence in the treatment because of the good results I've had with no side effects.

Other health problems have developed in the last six years, one being an arthritic flare-up in my wrists about one year ago. Returning to Iowa and Dr. Sinnott for the five day IV antibiotic treatment seemed to be what I needed, and that's what I did. Just recently I've wondered whether receiving regular IV antibiotics, maybe on a yearly basis, would have prevented this flare-up and another autoimmune disease (ITP, a blood disorder I developed about six years ago) from happening. Hindsight sheds light on present day situations, but follow-through is what matters. A few reasons I didn't go more often for the IV treatments was the distance involved in getting there and also when I'm feeling better I tend to get as minimal as I can with medication and treatment.

From this patient's point of view it was a step of faith for me to try this treatment. It gave me good and positive results, and many blessings, one being the people I've met there in Iowa and other patients from all over the country. I'm very grateful to have found a doctor with such wisdom, patience and willingness to try a simpler and more effective approach to treating rheumatoid arthritis. Thank-you Dr. Sinnott.

Second Corinthians 1:3-4
Blessed be the God and Father of our Lord Jesus Christ, the Father of mercies and God of all comforts; Who comforts us in all our affliction so that we may be able to comfort those who are in any affliction with the comfort with which we ourselves are comforted by God.

Roberta in California

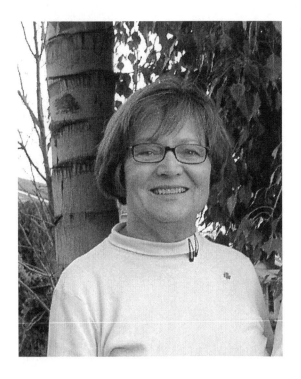

10

A Scleroderma Success Story*

My name is Dona Morris, and I have systemic scleroderma. The doctors believe it started in December 1988. I work for the Police Department in DeQueen, Arkansas. In mid-December we were involved in re-qualification exercises, and I fired a large number of rounds in my .357 revolver. We also dismantled our weapons, cleaned and reassembled them the same day. The next day my hands were painful and swollen, and I thought it was because we had fired and cleaned our guns on the same day - something we normally do not do. But the problem did not get any better. I couldn't turn the key to start my car without padding it with a tissue. I couldn't play my bass guitar.

My family doctor tried several anti-inflammatory drugs, all without relief. He began to suspect carpal tunnel syndrome as the pain was now all the way up my arms. I tried chiropractic treatments to see if they would help. In March of 1989, I had surgery on both wrists to relieve the pressure. The left hand improved but the right hand remained painful,

41

and I was unable to use it. Finally the doctor started giving me cortisone which was the only thing that relieved the pain. During this time I had a spell of severe fatigue which lasted ten days.

In October of 1989, I had surgery again on my right hand opening it into the palm where he found scar tissue binding the nerves. I had driven a school bus with a stick shift for years and believed that had caused the scar tissue and now my troubles would be over. How wrong I was!

About a week after the surgery I began to have joint pain which got progressively worse. My feet became swollen and it was painful to walk. Also, it felt like there was something in my throat even though I knew it couldn't be possible since I could still swallow several vitamins at a time. My family doctor was mystified but took a blood sample and gave me a one week supply of cortisone to give me some relief from the pain. From blood tests, my doctor thought I possibly had lupus and sent me to a rheumatologist where more tests were done. I was in a terrible state of mind having been in constant pain for a year now. I had always been a healthy person who ate right, took vitamins and walked two miles almost daily for several years. I couldn't understand why I was having all this trouble.

In January 1990 my fingers began to get contractures. A full muscle biopsy was done. Finally I was told I had limited scleroderma and given a prescription for [name brand] salsalate. It took a year to heal from that biopsy. I knew I did not have limited scleroderma because my throat was already affected. I asked my family doctor to send me to a diagnostic clinic in Temple, Texas for a second opinion. After numerous tests they said it was classic systemic scleroderma and that both my throat and lungs were affected. My skin was already darkened, and the skin around my mouth was tightening and limiting my ability to open my mouth. The skin all over my body was tightening.

I had already been in touch with the support group in New Castle, Pennsylvania and had read all their information. The doctor started me on penicillamine, ordered blood work every two or three weeks, and sent me home with instructions to return in June.

I couldn't tolerate the penicillamine, but when I went back the rheumatologist offered no other treatment. My skin was getting tighter, getting dressed was extremely difficult, and I couldn't brush my back teeth or bite a sandwich. Getting up from a chair was a struggle and I needed help. I went up and down the stairs like a baby would. The head of my bed was raised to prevent reflux into the esophagus. I couldn't fold my arms, reach up into a cabinet, or pick anything up off the floor. I couldn't sleep through the night because I hurt... hurt.... hurt. But worst of all was the sense of hopelessness. None of the doctors I had seen or read about knew what caused scleroderma or what to do for it. I was 55 years old and felt as I imagined someone 95 might feel. My husband was very supportive and patient with all my groanings, but he didn't know any more than I did about what to do.

It was through our minister's wife that I learned about someone in Bentonville, Arkansas who was taking an antibiotic for her scleroderma. She got the name of Dr. Brown's book and our librarians found a copy for me. I was reading it when I was sent to another rheumatologist. This doctor said the antibiotic treatment wasn't effective and intimated Dr. Brown was a quack, yet he had nothing to offer me.

My family doctor started me on the oral antibiotics in September of 1990, and in January of 1991 a doctor in Alabama prescribed the IV [name brand] clindamycin. The

IVs were administered by our state home care program. My skin was so hard they had difficulty starting the IV without blowing the vein since they had to push so hard to get through the skin. But as time went by my skin softened, the redness and soreness left my hands, and the open sores on my knuckles healed. Gradually the joint pain lessened and my feet began to feel normal. My throat problem improved. My range of motion has improved greatly, and I only have mild joint pain when the seasons are really unstable. I can get up from chairs normally, go up and down stairs normally, and even do floor exercises. The nurses who began my treatment were amazed at the difference in my condition as time went by.

I am still in treatment, although I am now with a doctor who has experience with this therapy. I don't know how much longer it will take, but it doesn't matter because it is working and I now have hope.

Update: April 15, 1999
I love to hear from people who are looking for a treatment that works, and I can certainly testify that Dr. Brown's treatment has worked for me. A portion of my story and a picture of me, taken in 1997 demonstrating my ability to climb a ladder and wash the outside windows, are included on page 305 of Henry Scammell's book The New Arthritis Breakthrough.

I have been in treatment since 1993 with Dr. John Sinnott of Ida Grove, Iowa who wrote one of the chapters in Dr. Thomas McPherson Brown's book, The Road Back. I continue to see Dr. Sinnott for a yearly checkup and blood tests. In June of 1997 we decided to try discontinuing my IV treatments since there had been no change in my condition or the blood tests for some time. However, Dr. Sinnott wanted me to continue the oral portion of my treatment

(100mg of minocycline twice a day, 3 days a week), which I did until last June 1998, when we cut that in half. My blood test in 1998 was still good after having been off the IVs for a year, and I fully expect it to be good this year since I'm feeling fine. I have good energy and really have no remaining symptoms of scleroderma, except my finger contractures, which Dr. Sinnott believes will be permanent. I do have better closure of both hands now as I continue to use them. I'm back to playing my big bass fiddle in our bluegrass band and having a great life thanks to God and Dr. Brown's treatment. I do expect to remain in Dr. Sinnott's care indefinitely to continue to monitor my condition.

Update: July 2001

I am continuing to do well and have just been to see Dr. Sinnott for my yearly blood test. The results were good. He still has me on half dosage of minocycline, but I feel that I would be just fine without any. I am able to do whatever I want to do, walk two miles a day, do strength training, take Line Dancing lessons, and feel fine.

Update May 2008

Dr. Sinnott and I agreed to stopping the oral meds. I have been off the oral meds for 6 months and have seen no changes in my condition. Additionally, beginning in 2005 I started going for blood tests every other year instead of yearly. All is still well.

DONA MORRIS
Phone U.S.A. 870-584-7678
tmorrisd@gmail.com

Special thanks to Stephen White for copyright permission in reprinting this modified story originally posted on rheumatic.org

Our Road Back

11

My RA Journey

In 2008 I was working at a Flower Shop designing a large funeral bouquet. My shoulder was in so much pain that after I got the bouquet done, I left and went to my doctor. He suggested a cortisone shot, which I agreed to although I knew nothing about it. For three days I felt so good, felt like I was 30 years old again (I was 62), but the fourth day was much different. I felt more like 90 years old. I couldn't get out of bed very well, and I was in a lot of pain. Went back to the doctor, and he tested me for RA, and that test came back negative. Couldn't figure out what I had. Finally after weeks of the doctor trying to figure it out, I got so bad my husband took me to the ER. That doctor took one look at my hands and said "You have rheumatoid arthritis."

Oh that hit me like a brick! All I could think of was a wonderful lady in our church that was so snarled up with RA for years, and I always said I sure won't want that disease. And now he said I had it. I was in total shock but still in pain. So he put me on prednisone, and we all know what that's like.

The ER doctor said I had a virus waiting to happen, and the cortisone shot just shook it up, and it gave me instant RA. WOW.. Right away I knew somehow I was going to find an answer to this disease. It was not crippling me up! For the next two years I was miserable. It took me eight months to get into a rheumatologist. He put me on methotrexate, and I finally got off the prednisone.

Had to keep going up with the meds so my stiffness would improve, but then along came the stomach problems, an ulcer, and the worst was the fatigue. I just wasn't getting that much better. Got around ok but slow. Go shopping, and I had to have a cart to lean on. I couldn't go down my stairs to do the laundry. I just felt like I was 90. I now had a new understanding of people in a rest home.

During this miserable time a friend of mine told me to go to Newsmax.com and get a book. It was written by Dr. David Brownstein. I did that, and it told me about another book: The Arthritis Breakthrough by Henry Scammell. And I read and read, and highlighted it. And the more I read, the more I knew this was my answer.

I had an appointment with my rhummy in April. At the end of January, I started taking myself off of the meds. I was going to get the antibiotic! I was so excited about it. I took my books all highlighted to the doctor's office. In comes a student nurse. I told her all about it, and showed her my highlights. She in turn told me "Your doctor knows all about that research at the University; he was on one of those studies." Oh, I was all excited for sure then. He'd understand and help me. Well.. that didn't happen. In he walks and never mentioned the study at the University where so many had been helped with antibiotics. Instead, he said NO!! Your skin will turn dark, and you don't want this. I said "YES I do" and he said "NO".. finally I said "It's my body, my pain… final answer.. I want the antibiotic!" He never said a word. He left, and a while later he walked in the door and handed me the prescription but with no extra instructions, just take 2 a day was on the bottle. He did say "Come back when it doesn't work." That was it. I've never been back. I had my book and *The Roadback Foundation* to help me with my answers. I learned fast about the herxing. And thanks to a wonderful lady I met online from Australia, I could always get answers.

In Henry Scammell's book, there's a chapter about Ida Grove, Iowa. OH, did my eyes open big!! IDA GROVE!! As a teenager I lived in the next town called Battle Creek. My dad was a pastor of a church there, and I was a cheerleader going to games in Ida Grove. Oh, that was like going home for me.

So, July of 2010 I went to Ida Grove. Stayed a week there and had the IV's. What loving, caring people Dr. Sinnott and his staff are! They said we may not notice any change immediately, but halfway through we would. At first, all I noticed was the copper taste, nothing else. I was still soaking my hands each morning in hot water due to the pain and stiffness. On Thursday morning, I woke up... NO PAIN!! No stiffness, no need to soak my hands. Now I had no more tears of pain.. just tears of joy. Praising the Lord for answers. The antibiotic worked and it worked so fast. Soon it will be spring of 2011, and I have three weddings booked... I can now go down my stairs... I have my floral studio down there.

Praise be to God and to the doctors that researched all this and dedicated their lives to helping so many. And thanks to Dr. Sinnott for all his years giving people hope, and their lives back... GOD BLESS YOU.

A.L.
South Dakota

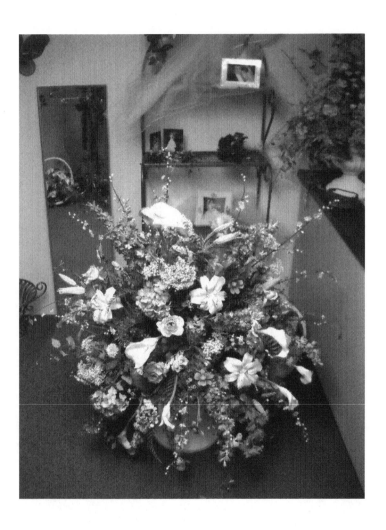

12

Road Back Journal

Nearly twenty years ago at age 19, I was diagnosed with a mild case of lupus. Unlike most of Dr. Sinnott's patients, I have taken only the oral antibiotics. The reason for this decision is because my health insurance will not cover this "experimental" treatment, therefore making it a financial impossibility. Below you will see a meager seven-day journal entry of my experience.

Day 1~ Fearful about a Herxheimer reaction, I started with just half the recommended dose of oral minocycline. Within an hour and a half I got the chills and my joints started hurting. The "brain fog" often described by lupus patients set in. Every joint that ever hurt in the past started hurting including my shins, forearms and rib cage. My fever was clocked at 100 degrees. As if that wasn't bad enough, it became hard to breathe because my blood pressure plummeted to 87/42. Walking up a flight of stairs exhausts me. Just three days ago I put in 45 minutes of jogging on the treadmill.

Day 2~ During the night my fever spiked. This morning however, I felt my symptoms lessen across the board. I took a [name brand] diphenhydramine and a morning nap. It helped. At 1pm I took only 50mg of minocycline, which was half the dose of yesterday. I would say that my reaction is only half of what it was yesterday. I took another 50 mg tonight. We will see how I do…

Day 3~ Much better.

Day 4~ No data recorded.

Day 5~ Almost to 100 mg of minocycline with food. The pharmacist was right, take it with food. I don't feel nauseated. My joints are swollen which is unusual for me.

Day 6~ The swelling continues. Odd pain under left knee. Will take 100 mg tonight. So far so good. Slight nausea. No fevers since day two.

Day 7~ I feel horrible after taking the 100 mg. Maybe if I remember to take the [name brand] diphenhydramine with it… My stomach bloats with the meds. Another headache. I have felt somewhat dizzy this week; I can't close my eyes when in the shower. I have also felt oddly calm, almost like I am on some good anti-anxiety medicine.

Unfortunately, I never recorded any more data after this point. Shortly after this period I did switch to doxycycline to avoid intense nausea. I still have to eat with the doxycycline or my stomach will get so upset that I have to lie down.

I believe I started the treatment in August of 2008. Six months later, for the first time since my diagnosis, I actually tested negative for my ANA. My physician said she has never seen anything like it. One year after that, I retested the

ANA and still negative! I have no reason to believe that it has spiked since then.

Now mind you, I still have sporadic joint pain and other bone pain. A bunion has also shown up on my left foot. I also sport a swollen knuckle on my left index finger. From time to time, I will swell up like I am having a horrible allergic reaction but it subsides after a day or two, just like it did prior to the treatment. While I still have minor annoyances, I can't help but to wonder what this treatment may be preventing. Even if nothing else, my negative ANA means less cumulative damage to my body in the long haul. Someday I hope to get the IV antibiotics. Perhaps then I will see an even further decrease in my symptoms.

Thank you Dr. Sinnott.

Gretchen Critelli
West Des Moines, Iowa

Our Road Back

13

Surviving CREST Scleroderma, Happy and Healthy

I received the diagnosis of CREST Scleroderma from doctors in 1996, at the age of 49. The diagnosis was totally unexpected. I had been referred to specialists with a pre-diagnosis of achalasia because of problems keeping food down after eating.

I had never heard of Scleroderma. The doctor did not explain the disease to me at that time. He made additional appointments for a second endoscopy, additional blood tests, and a stomach emptying study the following week.

My husband and I made a trip to our city library to see if we could find any information that might ease my sense of doom concerning the diagnosis. The information was hard to find and mostly in medical terms I did not understand. The hospital where my tests were scheduled was a drive of 90 miles from my home. Since my son lived in the same city as the hospital and my husband could not make the drive with me, my son took me to my appointments, and I spent the night after the tests at his home. My tests were completed and I was told to return to the hospital the following week for test results and to see a Rheumatologist. That night my son and I spent a lot of time talking about Scleroderma. We did a lot of research on his home computer that evening which really was an eye opening experience.

The following weekend, my son came home for a visit with a new computer for his Dad and I. He knew how important research would be for me to understand and deal with my diagnosis. Access to the internet and the realm of information available has had an enormous impact on our lives.

For the next few months, I frequently kept appointments with doctors specializing in Rheumatology and connective tissue diseases. I was placed on numerous costly drugs, many with adverse side affects. My pain levels increased, and my blood pressure continued to rise even though I took all medications as prescribed.

After several years following doctor's orders and joining several discussion groups on the internet, I miraculously discovered *The Road Back Foundation*. RBF recommended reading several books, so I made the trip back to our library where I found and read each book. Among those pages I discovered Dr. Sinnott and felt so blessed that he and I lived in the same state. I contacted his office and made an appointment to visit his clinic and start my Antibiotic Therapy in 2004.

My week in Ida Grove was probably the most relaxing and peaceful week I had spent in many years. I kept daily contact with my family by phone and received much encouragement from the staff at the hospital. The week went by very quickly and by weeks end, I really began to feel that I could look forward to a brighter future.

I continued my daily 200 mg of minocycline for the next five years with very good success. I worked everyday in my job as an Administrative Secretary, missing very little work due to illness. My family doctor was pleased with my good health and continued to care for me, although he wouldn't outright accept my Antibiotic Therapy as treatment for Scleroderma.

When my husband retired in late 2008, I asked Dr. Sinnott if I could try switching my prescription from minocycline to doxycycline due to loss of prescription coverage through my husband's work. He agreed to try the switch. I did not notice any difference for nearly a year on the doxycycline. As time went on, I began to notice familiar symptoms ever so slightly returning. I again contacted Dr. Sinnott and asked if I might benefit from intravenous AP therapy for a second time. I made an appointment and returned to Ida Grove in April 2010. After spending my week in Ida Grove, I returned to taking 200 mg minocycline daily.

I can honestly say that today I feel very good on a daily basis. I have retired at the age of 62 -- 14 years after my original diagnosis in 1996. My family and I fully agree that AP has possibly saved my life and given me a wonderful quality of life as well. My younger cousin died at 49 years of age with CREST.

Although I continue to take medications for high blood pressure, as well as proton pump inhibitors for prior damage to my esophagus, I feel very lucky and blessed to have found AP Therapy. I look forward to each and every day. I have been truly blessed knowing Dr. Sinnott and his staff since 2004.

If my story can help to answer just one question for someone diagnosed with a connective tissue disease, I will be grateful for the opportunity to help.

Sherry Boswell
Hollister, Missouri
ponytime66@hotmail.com

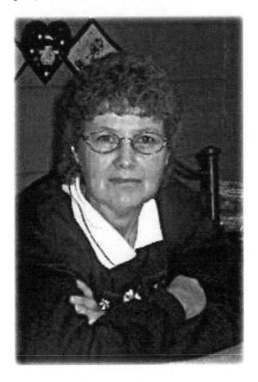

14

My Health Crisis

At the beginning of the summer of 2008 I began to have muscle pain, which I believed might be fibromyalgia. I attended physical therapy which helped some, but the pain would come back within a few days. I had some short-term relief from massage and acupuncture. After a few months I had some hip pain, and again went to physical therapy for that also, with temporary relief. Then the pain started to move around, to the shoulder, or the wrist. Fatigue was worsening throughout this time.

By the end of the summer, I started to have joint swelling and more pain. By October, I had stiffness which lasted about 22 hours of each day, and the joint swelling would move around – hips, feet, hands, etc. It eventually became so bad I had difficulty getting out of bed, couldn't get dressed without help, and had difficulty pulling up sheets at night, or even turning over. I couldn't open doors, food jars, and lost my fine and gross motor skills in my hands. If there had been a fire, I would not have been able to get out of the house through any exit, except the garage door by pushing the electronic opener. I could not slide or pull heavy doors or open the front door knob because I could not turn it. Some days I could not drive. For three months this continued, and I continued to work with the pain.

I tried some ibuprofen prescription strength, [name brand] acetaminophen, and then changed to aspirin. This didn't help the pain either. I had a visit with the doctor I work for, and he gave me a prescription for [name brand] celecoxib which didn't help either.

I suspected RA since I am a nurse practitioner, but resisted testing as the mind body connection is very strong. When people are confronted with hard evidence outside of their symptoms and sometimes (e.g. in cases of cancer where they may be asymptomatic) they become fatalistic and rapidly go downhill. Ignorance can be bliss. I found information on RA treatments such as another approach which I did try without success and I also found *The Road Back Foundation*. Over my treatment period I have worked with a volunteer who is a dedicated volunteer at *Road Back*. She gave me Dr. Sinnott's name and the good news of free phone consultations which I have been blessed to take advantage of several times for myself and for my own patients.

I saw a doctor that I worked with to confirm RA after finally taking the test that confirmed I had the Rheumatoid Factor in December 2008. This doctor was a rheumatologist before joining our integrative practice. He confirmed RA using a rheumatoid factor test, a physical exam, and symptoms. He started me on prednisone, [name brand] celecoxib (later changed to naproxen), and [name brand] hydroxy-chloroquine. I continued to be debilitated and in pain despite these treatments. I've also had steroid injections into some joints, with small or temporary relief.

This doctor has a long career as a rheumatologist and was willing to help me use the antibiotic protocol, but since our experience with this drug was nil, I went to an arthritis center in Riverside, California because they have been utilizing this therapy with good success for many years. At the center, Dr. L added clindamycin intravenously, which I was fortunate to obtain at work for no cost. This addition of monthly infusions has relieved me of the daily, crippling stiffness that kept me in bed most of the day. I did experience some worsening of symptoms called the Herxheimer, but overall I have had a decrease in swelling, joint pain, and stiffness. I am still struggling with fatigue and depression that accompanies chronic inflammation, but overall I am better. I do not have any joint deformity at this time.

Over the next year I continued with the [name brand] minocycline and clindamycin as well as making dietary changes. I was gluten free prior to getting RA, but added to the elimination list dairy, eggs, red meat and tomato sauce. Coffee, rare alcohol and rare sugar as well. These foods tend to exacerbate my arthritis sometimes within hours or the next day. I believe since eliminating these foods I have been able to reduce inflammation and speed up recovery time.

In January of 2009 I decided to reduce with the goal of eliminating the prednisone from my regimen. During the year I took this medicine, I lost half of my hair and now have cataracts.

During the summer of 2010, I continued in my quest for remission by improving my diet, reducing the frequency of my intravenous (sometimes intramuscular) doses of clindamycin, and I tapered off of my twice daily dose of naproxen. I no longer take this medication. I am now able to work part-time, ride a bike, and rarely have any stiffness at all. The only joint that is swollen is my joint in my middle finger on my right hand. I continued to exercise by going to a water aerobics class and riding my bike!

In the fall, I really felt that I was 90% close to being in remission. I added some [name brand] azithromycin twice a week because I had a long childhood history of strep throat even though my anti-streptolysin O titer was negative. This really improved the residual joint pain, and I almost felt normal. My middle finger joint finally went down. My last set of X-rays of my hands and feet this last December (2010) show no new erosions.

In my quest for remission, I have realized that not only is stress a mitigating factor, but so is past emotional hurts. I don't actively live in the past, but my past hurts are residing in my joints with my anger towards those who hurt me. I am working with my pastor to let these memories go, to free myself of my self-imposed prison. Being mad at those people who hurt me does nothing to them, but it does hurt me. I want out of my prison. I believe that the emotional component to RA is very strong, and maybe women struggle with this more than men.

I still have some aches and pains, but I am so pleased to be independent again. This treatment has been a real blessing to me. I am blessed to be able to help others with RA with a meaningful, almost no side effect treatment plan.

Lolita Hanks, RN, BSN, MS, FNP-C
Mom, Wife and Family Nurse Practitioner

15

My Journey to Ida Grove

My story is probably unlike others you will read in this book. My rheumatoid arthritis developed so quickly that I did not know what hit me. One month I was an energetic middle-aged college professor. The next month I was able to teach lessons which were mediocre at best and only from a seated position. I could not return to campus the following semester. I was both physically and emotionally devastated and had no idea why.

My first stop was a visit to my primary care physician. After many tests, including a CT scan of my brain, she decided to test for rheumatoid arthritis. BINGO!!

I was glad to finally have a diagnosis and to begin a medication regimen. However, my delight was short-lived as the drugs caused side effects which seemed worse than the disease. By this time it was necessary for me to use a wheelchair much of the time. My husband had to take a very early "retirement" to care for me.

Then I heard about Dr. Sinnott and did not know at the time that my life would be forever changed. I traveled to Ida Grove, skeptical but hopeful. What I remember most about my first visit is that Dr. Sinnott told me, "This is not a treatment for impatient people." So frankly, I did not expect much in the way of progress.

Those expectations were realized. The first series of antibiotic IVs in August 1999 did not change my condition at all. Four months later in December, Dr. Sinnott suggested repeating the process. I did, and again no noticeable difference in my condition. However, I continued on the oral antibiotic medication anyway.

By March 2000, I began to feel better. My husband noticed that my ability to walk was much improved. I began to get my life back! I remained on the oral antibiotics with occasional treatments of a single IV. Progress continued steadily.

When I sensed that Dr. Sinnott might retire, I searched for a doctor in my area that uses the same treatment. I located one, and I still take the oral antibiotic every day. I don't ever want to give it up.

The best indicator of my return to a "normal" life is that after I improved, my husband and I adopted a precious special needs newborn. I now have the best job I have ever had . . . a stay-at-home mom!

M.A.
USA

16

My Story About the Use of Antibiotic Therapy to Relieve the Symptoms of Rheumatoid Arthritis

HISTORY OF MY RA

My story starts in the winter of 2000. It was at this time I was informed of the fact that I had rheumatoid arthritis. It was not pleasant news; in fact it was rather discouraging. I had noticed that my big toe on my right foot had been hurting periodically. I didn't think anything of it, and after a while the discomfort went away. The next thing that happened was my right knee started to hurt. I felt it was something that had happened during wrestling practice and didn't think much about it, but the pain just kept getting worse. In the late winter the pain was more than I could take, so I went to see an orthopedic surgeon. After looking at my knee and taking an MRI it was determined that I had a torn cartilage. I went through same day arthroscopic surgery. This was to relieve my pain and help me get back to normal.

I scheduled surgery for early March, and as I came out of surgery I was informed by Dr. F_ that I did indeed have a torn cartilage, and he repaired the tear. However, he was surprised at how much pain I was in due to the tear. Within a few days my left knee started to hurt worse than my right knee. So it was back to Dr. F_, back to arthroscopic surgery, and back to the same post operative comments. A small tear but what a surprise at how much pain I was in.

After a couple of weeks my whole body started to hurt. My wrists, my ankles, my hips, my elbows, and even my knees again. I didn't want to tell anybody because I thought that I had something really bad, like Lou Gehrig's disease. After a couple of weeks of waking up in the morning and sitting on my steps for 10-15 minutes before I could put my socks on let alone tie my shoes, I decided that I had better tell my wife that something was wrong.

My family doctor, Dr. L_, asked me several questions and suspected that I might have something along the line of Lyme disease. He scheduled me to get my blood tested, and I rescheduled to see him the next week after the results were forwarded back to his office. He informed me that it was not Lyme disease but rather Rheumatoid Arthritis. I knew very little about RA but he gave me a 16-day cycle of prednisone, a type of steroid that is extremely efficient in relieving the pain but has some serious side effects. He informed me that I should schedule an appointment with a rheumatologist.

My experience with the rheumatologist turned out to be a total waste of time. I didn't feel comfortable with the doctor and what was prescribed did nothing to relieve any of the pain I had, in fact I knew that I was getting worse as the days went by. It was about this time that I called my friend, Kevin Dresser, and told him about my situation. He informed me that his mother, Laura Dresser, had RA and told me to call her. The phone call to her was extremely helpful since she knew exactly what I was going through, how I felt, and how discouraged I had become. She explained to me about life with RA and how she was at wits end until she discovered a Dr. John Sinnott in Ida Grove, Iowa. She explained how she tried everything and how after spending one day with Dr. Sinnott and getting on antibiotic treatment she was doing better both physically and mentally. She suggested that I skip everything and go see Dr. Sinnott. I called to schedule an appointment but never went through with it and canceled at the last minute.

Life went on and I started seeing my family doctor again. He had me taking methotrexate, [name brand] rofecoxib, and folic acid. I was doing fine until the fall of 2001 when my right knee had a large swelling which was determined to be a Baker's cyst. This cyst is caused by fluid being retained in the knee, and it needed to be drained or it could cause further damage. Dr. L_ scheduled an MRI and encouraged me to go back to Dr. F_ since he thought something was wrong and a specialist would be more helpful. Dr. F_ examined the MRI and noticed that I had fluid everywhere around my knee, above it, below it, and everywhere in between. He drained my knee with a syringe and explained to me that I needed to go back to a rheumatologist. I explained my experience to him, and he suggested that I see someone else.

So it was back to the rheumatologist. I liked this other rheumatologist much better; he kept me on methotrexate, and [name brand] rofecoxib but he added [name brand] hydroxychloroquine to the mix. I was also getting my blood checked one a month. I felt that things were going better but it wasn't long before I was back to feeling as bad as ever. I had an appointment with him in early July, and I informed him of my problems. I just wasn't doing better or even staying the same; I was getting worse. He explained to me that adding a new drug, [name brand] infliximab, to the mix should help.

Leaving his office I thought to myself, what the hell is going on! I wasn't getting better, and all I was doing was taking drug, after drug, after drug. Where would it end and even more importantly, how would it end? As soon as I got back home I called Laura Dresser again. She immediately asked how my appointment with Dr. Sinnott went. I explained that I never went, and I wanted to know if she was still feeling better or feeling worse. She was not only feeling better but seemed to be getting better all the time, even better than she was during our first conversation. She was taking a [name brand] rofecoxib everyday and taking minocycline twice a day on Monday, Wednesday, and Friday. No more blood work, no more dangerous drugs, and best of all no more feeling bad. At that point I decided that I would call Dr. Sinnott and schedule an appointment and see it through. My wife called, and I was scheduled for September 23-27, 2002.

MY TRIP TO IOWA

My trip to Iowa started on Sunday morning September 22, 2002. My wife and daughters started the morning by attending a cheerleading competition that day, and they needed to leave at 6:30 a.m. While getting up with my wife and helping my daughters we noticed that a skunk had just sprayed something in the immediate area. The something that got sprayed was our dog, so my morning started by going to the store to buy some vinegar. I washed the dog several times before it was time to head to the airport.

Arriving at the airport I was informed that my scheduled flight was overbooked, and I would be lucky to get out of Pittsburgh that day but I could take my chances. I decided to book my bags all the way through to Iowa, and I waited for the next plane to Pittsburgh. I took a seat on the flight and as soon as I landed in Pittsburgh, I rushed to the departing flight for Kansas City which was scheduled to leave at that exact minute. I moved as fast as I could through the terminal and was allowed to board the flight. So it was off to Kansas City. At Kansas City I waited for the flight to Cedar Rapids along with three other passengers and off we went. It was a rewarding flight since we flew over many areas that I grew up in, and it was really neat to see this area from the air. I arrived in Cedar Rapids and much to my surprise my bags did not; it would not be until the next day before my bags showed up. I spent the night at my parents' house and visited with my sisters and brother.

MONDAY SEPTEMBER 23

I got up and out of bed at around 7:30 in the morning. Sat down to eat a small breakfast with my dad, it was my usual breakfast in Iowa. A piece of toast with peanut butter spread on it washed down with a glass of milk. After eating and talking with my dad for a few minutes I jumped into the shower, put on a clean change of clothes and was off on my adventure to Ida Grove. I was to meet my Uncle Jim and Aunt Judy Gearhart in Denison, Iowa at a restaurant diner for lunch at 11:30. The trip across Iowa was very scenic at this time of the year; the leaves were turning their autumn colors but even better was the fact that all the farmers were in the fields harvesting their crops. I drove by miles and miles of corn and beans and witnessed many farmers driving big combines and unloading these same big combines. To me it was beautiful and brought back many wonderful childhood memories.

I arrived at the restaurant diner at 11:20 and waited for only a few minutes before Jim and Judy pulled up to greet me. The restaurant diner was a nice little diner and the people were quite friendly also. I ordered one of my favorites, pork tenderloin, and enjoyed visiting with Jim and Judy about life, the children, and my upcoming trip to see the doctor in Ida Grove. We finished eating and headed north for my visit. The country was very wide open in northern Iowa. It was quite a distance between towns and everything in between was corn and beans. We arrived in Ida Grove at approximately 1:15, unloaded at Dr. Sinnott's office, filled out some forms, and waited to be called back. At about 1:35 I was called back by a nurse and asked Jim, and more importantly, Judy to accompany me back to the room. The nurse took my blood pressure, recorded my heart beat, and weighed me in. She asked to sit and wait for the doctor.

Dr. John Sinnott then arrived on the scene. He seemed like a very nice and caring individual as he made introductions to everyone in the room. As soon as he finished, he sat down and starting asking me questions, how long, where did it hurt, does weather affect my condition, and other pertinent questions. After several minutes of questions he explained in great detail what he was going to do to treat my symptoms. He explained that arthritis is an infection and it can be handled with the use of antibiotics. This process would entail a week of twice daily intravenous treatments of antibiotics followed by indefinite use of oral antibiotics. He went on in greater detail that this process would not happen over night but would be more of a gradual process and that I would get worse before I felt better. With that he asked if I had any more questions, and then he sent me to the hospital (which just happened to be right across the street) for the start of my IV treatments.

The treatments started with the poking of my hand with a heparin lock, a semi-permanent device that connects with the IV, and taping the lock firmly in place. As soon as the lock was in place the treatments began; the IV contained [name brand] clindamycin. It took about 30 minutes for the IV to run its course at which time the nurse flushed the lock with saline and I was sent on my way only to be reminded to return in 6 hours for my second treatment of the day. At this point we left the hospital and headed to Randy and Cindy Ulmers' house in nearby Charter Oak, Iowa (30 miles).

Arriving at the Ulmers' was a somewhat unusual situation since we had never really met. It was obvious from the start that they were very nice people, and I immediately felt comfortable as they welcomed me into their house. Randy is employed at a meat products supplier in Denison and Cindy is a beautician who worked out of her home. They had two children Tanner, who was a freshman at a local college in Cedar Rapids, Iowa and Ivy, who was a student at the local high school which just happened to be right down the block. We had a nice dinner along with Jim, Judy, Tanner, Ivy, Randy, Cindy, and Ina (Randy and Judy's mom) and it just happened to be Ivy's birthday so we sang her "Happy Birthday", had cake and ice cream, and visited.

I left to go back for my second IV treatment at 8:30, but before I left I made plans with Jim and Judy for lunch on Tuesday at the restaurant diner in Denison. The second treatment went smooth, hooking up the IV followed by the flush of saline and I was done for day one. I was back at the Ulmers' around 10:00. I watched a little TV with Cindy and Ivy and headed upstairs to call it a night.

TUESDAY SEPTEMBER 24

I awoke the next morning at approximately 8:00 and decided to go for a nice bike ride, although I didn't really know for sure where I was going. I rode around town before venturing out in the country and riding for around 30 minutes at which time I headed back and did some exercises and stretching. After 15 minutes of exercise I took a shower and headed for my first IV treatment of the day. The trip to Ida Grove was very relaxing, gentle rolling hills, and corn fields as far as the eye can see. I arrived at the hospital and took my place in the little room that is designated for IV patients. The process was the same as the day before. Greetings by the nurse, hooking me up for 25-30 minutes, followed by the saline flush.

I left the hospital, filled the car with gas, and headed for Denison (27 miles) for a lunch date with Jim, Judy and Ina. Following lunch we headed to Ina's house to visit about things and passed the day away. A couple of hours passed by rather quickly and it was time to return for the next treatment. While heading back I decided that I needed to record this visit to Iowa, so I stopped at the store in Denison, purchased a camera, and was again on my way. I stopped by the hospital and did my fourth IV treatment, the process took about 30 minutes followed by a saline flush, and I was on my way to Charter Oak for the night. I arrived at the Ulmers' house at about 5:15, ate a nice dinner, and went upstairs and fell asleep at 7:30.

WEDNESDAY SEPTEMBER 25, 2002

I awoke at 8:00 and felt quite refreshed after the 12 hours of sleep from the night before; I think I was just wiped out from the entire ordeal of travel by air and car, the IV treatments, and being away from home. I put on my workout clothes and went for a nice bike ride followed by exercises. I cleaned up and headed to Ida Grove for my fifth IV treatment and finished with the treatment at 10:30. After the treatment I drove around town and stopped at the post office to mail some letters. I then walked across the street to call several people, including my mom, Tim Flynn, Laura Dresser, and Fairview High School. After the phone calls were finished I decided it was time to eat so I headed downtown and found a nice little restaurant and ate lunch. They had a buffet for lunch and I ate my fair share, the food was very good, and the atmosphere was relaxing. As I finished I decided to go to the library and relax until my next IV treatment.

While relaxing in the library I met a nurse from the hospital. She was a very nice lady who took me all around town and showed me all the sights including a bike/walking trail around the town, the Ida Grove – Battle Creek High School, the country club, all the industries in town, and finally she took me to Dr. Sinnott's house. I really enjoyed the tour and it reinforces the fact that the Midwest people are some of the friendliest and nicest in the U.S. After the tour she took me back to the library. I stayed until it closed, and then I returned to the hospital for my IV treatment. After the IV treatment I returned to Charter Oak ate a nice dinner and watched "We Were Soldiers" with Randy, Ivy, and Ivy's boyfriend from Denison, Iowa who seemed like a nice young man. After the movie I called it a night at around 10:30 p.m.

THURSDAY SEPTEMBER 26, 2002
I awoke at 8:00 and talked to my wife Kathy on the phone; everything was good back in Pennsylvania. When I was finished with the phone call I went for a real nice bike ride out in the country south of town, it was a nice ride which was very relaxing. I went for my IV treatment at 10:15 and finished about 10:45. I drove around and took several pictures of the sights from the day before. I ate lunch at a sandwich shop; while there some State Police came in and talked about a bank hold-up right across the state line in North Grand Fork, Nebraska earlier in the day.

I then traveled back to the library and read until 4:00 at which time I left to visit Don Knop. Don is the individual who was first diagnosed with rheumatoid arthritis in the mid seventies. He traveled to Dr. Brown's office in Washington, D.C. and brought back the antibiotic therapy to in Ida Grove, Iowa. Don said if it was not for Dr. Brown and Dr.

Sinnott he would be in a wheelchair or dead by now. I closed the conversation with Don and headed to the hospital for my IV treatment. The IV would not flow so they had to hook a pump to it to get it to flow into my body; the whole process took over an hour. I headed back to the Charter Oak and watched the girls' volleyball game against Manning. It was an exciting game and the school had a nice supply of supportive fans. I met the principal of the school and scheduled a visit with him the next day. I went back to Ulmers' for a late diner and went to bed in anticipation of the upcoming day.

FRIDAY SEPTEMBER 27, 2002

I set the alarm for 5:00 am so I could get an early start with everything and arrive at my parents' house back in Ely before dark. I arrived at the hospital to start my IV treatment at 5:30 and finished with the treatment at 6:10 am, and it was still dark outside so I went back out to my car and took a nap until it was daylight, right around 7:00. At this point I drove down to the library parked the car and unloaded the bike and started off on my ride.

Ida Grove has a beautiful bike trail around town and it even has a part of the trail that leads out into Morehead Park. I took off on my bike and headed right out to the trail that leads to the park. As soon as I arrived in the park I noticed that some cows had escaped the fence and were all over the park. I pedaled slowly through the cows and headed out into the nature trails. What a wonderful ride; I saw several deer, a flock of turkeys, some squirrels and rabbits, and more misplaced cows. I headed back into town and pedaled slowly just enjoying the sights.

I loaded the bike after the ride and headed back to the hospital for the final IV treatment and chance to discuss everything with Dr. Sinnott. I told him how pleased I was with the hospitality of everyone. He told me the process would take time and that I would most likely get worse before I got better. He told me to call back in a couple of months, and he would change my medication if needed and to just to let him know how things were going. He left, and I was once again hooked up to the IV for the tenth and final time of this trip. The IV wouldn't take so I had to be hooked up to the pump. The process took about an hour and as soon as they finished I had the lock removed from the top of my hand. I thanked everyone and was on my way to Charter Oak to clean up and say good-bye to the Ulmers'. They were extremely friendly and made me feel extremely welcome from the moment I first met them. I then walked down to the local high School and had a short visit with the principal. He gave me a nice tour of the building handed me some school papers to review, and I was on my way.

It was nice to be finished with the whole process, and I was glad to be heading home. The trip home was nice since the weather was beautiful, and the scenery was harvest time with tractors and combines working the fields and trucks hauling grain all over the place.

When I arrived in Cedar Rapids, I stopped by the local pharmacy to fill my first prescription. My sister Michelle works there and I just wanted to explain the whole week long process to her. She invited me to come along with her family that night to watch the local high school football game. That weekend I returned to Pennsylvania and within a week I started to feel much better. After a month, I felt real good and even considered myself back to normal.

November 1, 2002

It has been three months since my visit to Iowa. I feel so much better than before I went; I can't begin to explain the difference. Before I was hardly able to get up and walk to the bathroom or down the steps. Jogging was out of the question. I can do anything I want today: swimming, jogging, wrestling, lifting weights, biking, you name it. I don't feel perfect but I'm close, and I'm normal. The best part is I feel a little better each and every day. The only time I notice a problem is when a change of weather is coming through, but the bad feeling is only temporary. I feel that I owe many thanks to many different people. If not for these people I don't know where I would be right now. Thank you to Laura Dresser, my wife Kathy, Jim and Judy Gearhart, Randy and Cindy Ulmer, my mom and dad, all the nurses at the hospital and Dr. John Sinnott. All of you people have helped me reclaim my life from this horrible disease.

May 15, 2003

At this point in time everything is going very well in my life. I've been working out six days a week and haven't noticed any problems whatsoever. I've been eating normal, and I'm still taking two minocyclines a day and one [name brand] rofecoxib. I have also been taking three to four fish oil capsules everyday; I don't know if they help but they can't hurt. It has been really wonderful feeling normal again. I now look forward to the future, and again I'm feeling a little bit better each and every day while I'm on this treatment.

March 23, 2004

I just returned from the National Wrestling Tournament in St. Louis, Missouri. Again, I feel like a normal person. I went to workout everyday while in St. Louis: running around the Arch and Mississippi Rivers, riding the exercise bikes, and drilling with our heavyweight who was a national qualifier. It is so nice to be able to do these things again.

I workout every morning at school running, lifting weights, swimming, and biking during warmer weather and feel great doing it. I am still taking [name brand] rofecoxib, minocycline, a multi-vitamin, and fish oil every day. I don't really watch my diet too much; I eat as much as I want when I want. I look forward to the future and feel that this treatment is the best thing for me. I don't want to ever feel like I did before I went to Iowa in the fall of 2002.

I obtained the antibiotic protocol which was downloaded from the internet at *www.roadback.org*. They also have Dr. Sinnott's contact information.

October 2007

Things are really going well for me as I write this paragraph updating my story. Right now I take a minocycline about three times per week, a [name brand] celecoxib about once a week, and fish oil about every other day. I feel really good and just ran the Race Around Erie, which was a 15 km or 9.32 miles and won my age group.

Dr. Michael J. Hahesy, Ed.D

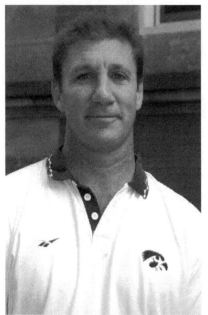

Photo Courtesy of
Edinboro University of Pennsylvania

17

30 Years of Scleroderma
Now in Reversal

I've had Scleroderma (SD) since age 3.5 (when the first signs of Raynaud's appeared) which was possibly triggered either by cytomegalovirus (CMV) or a strep infection I had six months prior. I was diagnosed for the first time at age six and am 34 years old now. I have a very mild case of SD despite it being diffuse which I attribute to regular use of tetracycline and other antibiotics prescribed by my mum (an MD) throughout my childhood when combating my frequent strep infections. My other lab results are absolutely normal, and I have no problems with my internal organs whatsoever. I live a full life, and my discomfort is only in my hands/fingers as they have always been. In April 2010, it was confirmed that I had diffuse scleroderma. I've been on the H_ Protocol since June 2010.

Having had this disease for over 30 years, I was so lucky not to develop any internal organ involvement. Only my external muscles were affected by becoming harder and tighter; my ligaments also hardened. My skin overall became tighter but did not restrict my movements in any way. My hands were effected by Raynaud's the worst. I have hard hands, all the fingertips had pitting scars, both index fingers are slightly deformed but none of my fingers are bent or crooked, and I can use my hands easily, e.g. when typing, sewing (but not without some discomfort). My face was also affected. My features changed. I grew thinner lips, nose, rounder eyes, not able to crease my forehead (but able to frown). I have microstoma (small mouth), crowding teeth, and receding gums around two teeth (all as a result of Scleroderma). Also, my entire skin is of permanently bronze-tanned colour with a reddish tint. All these changes occurred between ages 5 and 11 after which there was stability and with the beginning of my treatment, subtle improvements.

Soon I will be going through a series of routine tests which I do every three months to check my disease status and any damage from antibiotic use to my liver/kidneys. My last check up was in January, and it showed that for the first time (every since I started checking it in 2005) my ANA was negative, although my anti-Scl-70 antibodies were still positive but down from over 200 to 119.9 (normal is below 25). The first time I checked my anti-Scl-70 antibodies was in April 2010 before I started AP. It was 116 but went up to over 200. Now that the ANA is negative, it went down again. Besides this, I also had very subtle almost unnoticeable changes such as skin and tissue softening and healing of old fingertip ulcers... But I'll be able to discuss this with more confidence after I get my antibodies re-checked in April during my routine lab testing.

Update June 8, 2011
I received all my test results today. My ANA is STILL negative(!) although the anti-Scl-70 is still positive. I just spoke to Dr. Sinnott, and he explained how to read these

results. Basically, it's a very good sign my ANA stayed negative and that the anti-Scl-70 antibodies have no significant value for the purpose of treatment and evaluation. They are part of me so may not change. ANA, on the other hand, is an indicator of inflammation from SD, and it being negative is all that matters plus how I generally feel, and I feel very good. In fact, in one year since I started AP, I had no sickness whatsoever.

I also have to mention I take lots of various supplements and try to follow a nutritional plan as recommended by Dr. M_. I improved in many other areas as well which may or may not be connected to [brand name] minocycline - my polycystic ovarian syndrome (PCOS) is gone, all hormones are totally perfect. In fact, my testosterone is quite low now and my periods are painless and exactly on time.

In addition to [brand name] minocycline (100 mg BID), I also take systemic enzymes to reduce my fibrinogen levels which is responsible for sticky blood and poor circulation in rheumatoid patients. The systemic enzymes help dissolve fibrous tissue thus softening them in all parts of the body and reduce fibrinogen in the blood, in my case from 460 to 415 with normal being less than 350. By increasing my dose, I hope to achieve further reduction which should improve my blood circulation to lessen the Raynaud's attacks. Another drug I'm taking is LDN (low dose naltrexone), 4.5 mg - not sure how it helps, but I will continue it for a while longer (it must be helping though).

So all these meds have kept me in perfect health. As I mentioned above, I also take carefully selected vitamins and supplements, eat healthy, avoid processed foods, minimum starch, carbohydrates and gluten, but plenty of organic food, veggies (raw or lightly steamed), etc. In accordance to my nutritional type, I eat a lot of protein foods, including organic grass fed, free range red meats with all its fat on, other high purine meats, oily fish and make sure my meat is not overcooked or charred. I use a lot of extra virgin olive oil for cold cooking and organic virgin coconut oil and organic ghee (clarified butter) exclusively for hot cooking (my cholesterol is ideal). Unfortunately, with two small kids and work, I'm still not able to find time for exercise, though. My mum has kept me away from unhealthy foods all my life, and I never had a real sweet tooth which is one of the reasons why my disease is so mild! How and what you eat is really very important!

I arrived at this treatment plan independently from my health advisor. Books and the Internet were my only advisors. If I left it to doctors I came across, I would either be on no treatment plan of any sort or on a daily dose of an antimalarial drug [brand name] hydroxychloroquine sulfate and calcium channel blocks.

However, doctors did something good for me when I was nine which I attribute to my well being now. When I was nine, I developed rheumatic fever. I had fleeting arthritis, severe angioedema (normally triggered by viral infections), and low grade fever. It was the result of recurrent strep infections, and it started to affect my heart (I had arrhythmia). I was admitted to a pediatric hospital's rheumatic ward and stayed there for one month on a course of vitamins and penicillin. When the rheumatic fever was under control, I was transferred to ENT (Ear, Nose, Throat: otolaryngology) for tonsillectomy. After this, I stopped having such frequent strep infections. Angioedema attacks due to viral infections gradually decreased, my immunity grew stronger, and any developments of my SD had also stopped. In fact, as I hit puberty I started to get well at an increasing speed and became almost normal by age 17-18. At age 17-18, I underwent regular sessions of acupuncture which greatly softened my facial skin. I took courses of treatment with ginseng extract for 3-4 years, had several cleansing enemas after which my immunity grew much stronger and all the angioedema attacks ceased completely. My complete heart function tests in 2010 revealed absolutely no signs of past rheumatic fever which I was told was due to correctly designed and administered treatment.

I was underweight, almost anorexic between ages 5 and 18. I had a poor appetite and looked sickly, but I was full of energy and had no malabsorption issues. People used to joke that I moved so much I must burn whatever little I ate, and my mum should feed me better. But I just could not eat and did not want to eat. Due to my physique, I was selected for acrobatic lessons at school and was able to attain junior levels between ages 7 and 11. I dropped sports due to the damage it was doing to my spine and switched to ballroom and disco dancing lessons which I continued till I was 14. Then I dropped all these since I had to concentrate on my studies. This shows that despite my condition, I was able to live a full life all my life and even engage in sports involving flexibility.

Another important aspect I would like to mention is the importance of one's mental state when dealing with SD. My family never told me I have a life threatening disease. It was never discussed like that in out family. Officially, all I "had" was "Raynaud's phenomenon". My mum managed to hide her fears from me and always said I had nothing serious and it will go away (she knew how bad SD can be as she is an anesthesiologist physician herself). I lived strongly believing in that. And every time my mum gave me an herbal treatment, a cleansing enema, sent me to acupuncture or physiotherapy, it was officially just for my Raynaud's and my weak immunity! She had an agreement with all the therapists, and they never mentioned my disease to me either. I lived in complete oblivion up until I got pregnant. However, all these years my mum always closely watched any medical procedures I underwent and ensured my heart is double checked before administering any anesthesia (For example, my wisdom teeth were removed under general anesthesia. They couldn't do it at the dentist due to microstoma from SD and had to send me to hospital).

I have to say I developed an interest in medicine and even wanted to become a doctor myself like many of my family members, but life's circumstances turned me towards engineering school instead. However, I maintained my interest in medicine. I read up a lot including about Raynaud's phenomenon and did come across Scleroderma. Every time I had a finger inflammation I'd ask my mum if it was possible I have SD and she'd say "No, you don't have it!" My finger would get well in one month maximum, and I kept believing her because I was nowhere near as bad as they were describing in the books and on the Internet, but I started to grow suspicious that what I have is more than just the primary Raynaud's. I dug more into the Internet and what I found made me ask for ANA testing at the routine antenatal appointment. This was in 2005. My test came back positive. No titres, no pattern, just positive! Because my first two pregnancies spontaneously aborted, I got checked up for Lupus and other conditions which may cause miscarriages, including genetic testing but it all came back negative. I also tested positive for CMV antibodies (known to cause SD). All I had to think about was the dreadful SCLERODERMA!

I tried not to think about it, and it was easy since they discovered I had PCOS in 2003 which could mean I may have difficulty conceiving. This became my number one priority. However, my PCOS was not "normal". It was and wasn't there. I had some markers of PCOS but not really the full picture of it. I was not overweight, I had no acne or excessive facial hair, my hormonal status was not fully representing the classic PCOS picture. And despite the diagnosis, I never missed periods, had at least 11 normal (but very painful) periods every year and got pregnant easily which is not compatible with the PCOS diagnosis either. I easily became pregnant the third time (again with PCOS against all the odds) in 2006 and went on with the pregnancy normally. In fact, I sailed though it. No morning sickness or other side effects. My tummy grew nicely, the baby was of normal size (i.e. no growth retardation which is possible in SD patients), my skin got softer (experienced during pregnancy by SD patients). My tummy was soft, and by this time I was sure I had SD because as I was intrigued and continued digging deeper, I went to see a rheumatologist to get a diagnosis.

Mum came with me (as always). The doctor told me he doesn't even need to do any tests to tell me I have it. He only needs to look into my face to know I do. He quickly checked me over and said: "Go home and be happy you will not have wrinkles!" He refused to check the type of SD I have saying: "Why do you need to know? It doesn't make any difference for us as we are only interested in symptoms you show which may vary from person to person and from one SD type to another. So when you have any symptoms come back to me!" I was angry at him. At the time I saw him I was five months pregnant. He told me to come back after the delivery and go through some extensive tests such as lung capacity test, echocardiogram, stress ECG. He said I would need calcium channel blockers for my Raynaud's which I could take after the baby. I did not go back to him. I did not want to take any drugs.

My obstetrician put me on low dose aspirin and monitored me for any side effects from SD. We planned a C-section because of the SD, and it was planned just a day before my due date (as per my request), and my doctor kept smiling that she would be surprised if I carried it to full term (due to my SD). And she was right – I did not! As expected with SD patients, I had premature membrane rupture and ended up having an emergency C-section at 36 weeks plus one day (this happened when we were dining at an Italian restaurant, so from there we went straight home, picked up my bags and straight to the hospital). By now I was sure I had SD but I could not care less – I was having a baby. I had the most healthiest and beautiful little girl, weight higher than usual for her gestational age and despite her being slightly premature, she was in perfect health, very strong and we went home after three days. I was a normal mum, she was a normal baby. Even if I had SD I knew I was one of the lucky ones! My girl grew perfectly, and I recovered very soon after the C-section, was able to nurse for nine months, and did not think of SD too much. But it did lurk in the back of my mind. However, I stayed positive. I was even happy to have SD because thanks to that, my wounds healed really quickly, and I had no stretch marks of any sort!

When my daughter was 14 months old, I decided to try for number two and because I "had" PCOS, I thought I may have a couple of miscarriages again so why waste time? Do it now. And we got pregnant immediately. This made me think I'm either very lucky or there is something wrong with my PCOS diagnosis, or maybe my PCOS is the result of SD so it's not real but just a pseudo-PCOS caused by SD. I sailed through my second pregnancy, too. This time the baby was bigger and full term. I went into a planned C-section, had a large baby (What? SD? What SD? If I had SD he could not grow so nicely inside me and be 7.5 lbs at birth!) That's how I started to think now!

So, positive thinking, or not even thinking you have SD really helps. It keeps you from falling into despair and negative thinking thus preventing your disease from taking over and leading you down a bad course. You think positive and the disease treats you well. You don't think of it, and it doesn't bother you. If you fall into its claws, you will become its victim! I believed in this and even when I did not think I had SD, I took my Raynaud's as a reminder to be a "good girl." "If I'm bad the Raynaud's will become worse" I thought to myself and stayed a positive person trying not to upset other people too much and not to hold any grudges. Forgive, ask for forgiveness, and move on positively. It seems to surely work for me.

I enjoyed being free of any concerns about SD but not for long. When my son was six months old, I started to notice that my inflamed fingers wouldn't get better (luckily I do not have calcinosis but only inflaming, pitting scars at my fingertips). Before, they used to heal in 1-1.5 months max, but now they lasted for over two years... My right thumb became slightly stiff. All that was very painful and I survived only with help of a moisturiser! I had many horrible nights when all I wanted to do was to chop my fingers off, so unbearable was the pain at times! The moisturiser I used was really helpful though, and I went through dozens of tubs in those 2.5 years!

This is when I started digging again, and this time (with confidence I have SD) I told my mum, but she still wouldn't admit it. However, she listened to my findings very carefully. When I found out about the AP, I told her and she supported me. But first I wanted to make sure I have SD through blood tests and what type I have. In 2010, I had my first (known to me) official diagnosis of diffuse scleroderma, with ANA and anti-Scl-70 tests were positive. The doctor who ordered the test was surprised I had it (due to my previous annoying experience, I did not go to a rheumatologist but a dermatologist). He told me to watch my condition and check myself out if anything starts going wrong. He did not prescribe any meds to me or refer me to a rheumatologist as he believed I'm totally fine.

I now needed to find somebody who would prescribe the antibiotics I needed for AP. First I decided to try a rheumatologist again. She was educated at UCLA and knew about AP very well. She checked me over (much better than the first one I visited four years ago), sent me for lung, heart and some other tests and when the results came back absolutely perfect she said I will probably get better than worse from now on. However since she did not believe in AP, she would not prescribe any antibiotics for me. But because I was doing fine, she would allow me to experiment with AP myself without her involvement. If I have a more serious case of SD, she would put me on the normal drugs they use in such cases. She told me the name of the tetracycline antibiotic I could use and the dosage and told me to do routine blood tests to monitor the antibiotic's effect on me (She meant mainly from the side effect point of view, not curing point of view).

I did not want to take the generic antibiotic since I read the name brand was more effective for SD patients. That antibiotic was not available in the UAE so I had to find a physician who would agree to prescribe me the antibiotic which is not available in the UAE. I went to a GP clinic to see a doctor whose specialty was Infectious Diseases. Just what I needed! I told him about the AP, the causes of SD, and the infectious theory. He listened carefully and agreed to help as long as I lead him through the theoretical part since he did not have time to read it all but would trust me since he found me very adept at medicine. He also knew I was in contact with Dr. Sinnot by this time and that he is experienced, and I will get all treatment instructions from him so he only had to prescribe me the drug in the dosage Dr. Sinnot advises and do routine tests Dr. Sinnott recommends to check for treatment progress and antibiotic side effects.

Since I had my second son (both my children were delivered by C-section only due to limited tissue preventing normal delivery), I noticed my right hand starting to get worse. The fingertip pitting scars inflamed on two fingers and wouldn't heal for 2+ years when previously the longest it wouldn't heal was for two months. My right thumb became slightly stiff. All that was very painful!

I have to say that after one year into my treatment, all my ulcers are under control now; no new inflammations besides the tip of my right big toe being slightly more sensitive (but not really getting worse). I can see overall softening in my body, possibly from combination of [brand name] minocycline with systemic enzymes playing a greater role here as well.

The tip of my nose is softer, my ears are softer, lips stretch better. My skin is also much softer and so are my muscles. I feel my joints are looser (never realized they were stiff before.. this is what I grew up with and didn't know any better!), my ligaments are looser. I even wobble when I walk now! It's like I'm getting to know my body as it should have been. Also, I don't get frozen shoulders as much so do not require frequent back massages anymore (to my husband's great relief!). My thumb is not getting worse but it's still harder to bend than the other fingers. I still get Raynaud's. I know it mainly happens when I'm hungry, do not eat well, or if it's chilly or cold for a long period of time. I notice I get the attacks when it's below 23-22°C.

So I now know better what to do or not to do in order to prevent the attack or quickly reverse it. Dr. Sinnott says the attacks may continue happening but maybe with less frequency. However, due to the long history of my disease, the damage may be irreversible. I should take care not to let it worsen and continue taking minocycline for the rest of my life and eating right for my nutritional type, providing my body with the correct fuel it needs for keeping my body warm.

I am very thankful to my mum and how she protected me from this disease as a child and did not fall into despair, but instead curing me with alternative methods, supporting me and giving me courage when needed. She was once ready to cut a hole in my trachea one night when I was 10 or 11 during an angioedema attack threatening to become anaphylactic shock. These were the worst times in the USSR; medicine was at a downfall in Azerbaijan, ambulance service was not reliable. She filled a syringe with antihistamine, and with the syringe in one hand and the scalpel in the other, she explained to me that if the injection didn't work she would need to make a hole in my neck and put a rubber tube in it to allow me to breath until medics arrive. I had to be brave, so I agreed. But thankfully the injection worked quickly!

She is such a brave woman, and I owe her a lot for my life, my success, and for making me interested in medicine so that I am able to take control of my own hands and help myself. I am now helping her to combat her diabetes. My dad has passed away, but he was a great support for me, too. He brought me up as a fighter, teaching me to face challenges, not to give up easily, persevere and triumph. He supported my mum in her method of protecting me. He supported my interest in medicine (but was happy when I ended up an engineer just like him and in his field, too). My dad would be very proud of me now (as is my mum) who also believe that:

Nothing is impossible, persistence and education pay back generously

Aynur
Baku, Azerbijan

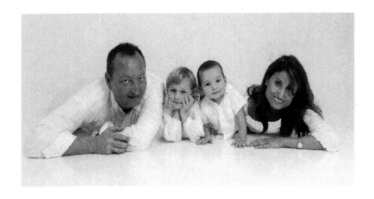

Our Road Back

Abbreviations

ANA	antinuclear antibody
anti-Scl-70	anti-topoisomerase I antibody
AP	antibiotic protocol
ASAP	as soon as possible
BID	twice a day
°C	Celsius
C-section	Caesarean section
CMV	cytomegalovirus
CPAP	continuous positive airway pressure
CREST	calcinosis, Raynaud's phenomenon, esophageal dysmotility, sclerodactyly, telangiectasia (acronym for limited form of scleroderma)
DT	delirium tremens
ECG	electrocardiogram, EKG
ER	emergency room
GP	General Practitioner
IV	intravenous
lbs	pounds
LDN	low dose naltrexone
LD	Lyme disease
MD	Medical Doctor
meds	medications
mg	milligram
MRI	magnetic resonance imaging
PCOS	polycystic ovarian syndrome
PMR	polymyalgia rheumatica
RBF	Road Back Foundation
rhummy	rheumatologist
SD	scleroderma
sed	sedimentation
TMJ	temporomandibular joint
UAE	United Arab Emirates
UCLA	University of California, Los Angeles
USSR	Union of Soviet Socialist Republics
wk	week

Our Road Back

John S. Sinnott, DO

Dr. Sinnott is a semi-retired physician who has been practicing medicine in Ida Grove, Iowa for over 40 years and is a member of the American Osteopathic Association. His special interest is in the use of antibiotic treatment for rheumatoid arthritis and other connective tissue diseases. Dr. Sinnott has dedicated much of his time to continuing the works of the late Thomas McPherson Brown, MD. He and his beautiful wife Lenee' enjoy relaxing on the family winery, as well as spending time with their new grandchildren... twins!

https://sites.google.com/site/johnssinnottdo/

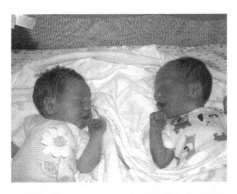

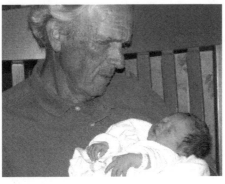

Our Road Back

Dr. Yang's Family Care

Dr. Yang's Family Care is a 501(c)(3), non-profit medical practice located in Santee, California dedicated to providing integrated, comprehensive, quality medical services, including continuing the works of the late Thomas McPherson Brown, MD.

Therese Yang, MD is the Medical Director and President of Dr. Yang's Family Care. She is board certified by the American Academy of Family Physicians with over 20 years of experience. After graduating from the University of Michigan, she spent four years studying the specialty of Family Practice, is happily married, and is raising her four beautiful children in southern California.

Working in two community clinics and a private practice, as well as volunteering on several boards, inspired Dr. Yang to start this non-profit office in 1997. Her mission is to provide integrated, quality medical care, especially to those who are not receiving the care they need elsewhere. A dedicated, multi-talented team and community support her towards achieving their goal.

http://dyfc.org/dryang.htm

Our Road Back

Hanna Rhee, MD

Dr. Rhee is a primary care provider and a member of the American Academy of Family Physicians. She received her Bachelor of Sciences Degree in Biological Sciences from the University of California at Irvine and went on to obtain her Medical Degree from the University of South Florida College of Medicine then medical internship and postgraduate training at the University of Colorado Hospital in Denver.

Dr. Rhee traveled extensively to research the growing field of immunoneuropsychiatry involving rheumatoid arthritis, Lyme disease, and Gulf War Illnesses. From Hawai'i, she voyaged to Iowa and studied the works of the late Thomas McPherson Brown, MD and his use of antibiotic therapies in arthritic patients. Dr. Rhee then trained in a Lyme disease endemic region of New York to better care for patients with persistent illness. Landmark studies at the genetic level by Garth L. Nicolson, PhD have provided her with the evidence-based research to better understand and care for our Gulf War veterans. She currently maintains a private practice in Carlsbad, California and continues to investigate current treatment options, write books, and publish research findings. Dr. Rhee is committed to continuing the works of Dr. Brown, treating persistent Lyme disease, and caring for our Gulf War heroes in the context of immunoneuropsychiatry.

www.hannarhee.com

Our Road Back

Made in the USA
Middletown, DE
02 September 2019